Strep Throat Demystified: Doctor's Secret Guide

Dr. Ankita Kashyap and Prof. Krishna N. Sharma

Published by Virtued Press, 2023.

While every precaution has been taken in the preparation of this book, the publisher assumes no responsibility for errors or omissions, or for damages resulting from the use of the information contained herein.

STREP THROAT DEMYSTIFIED: DOCTOR'S SECRET GUIDE

First edition. September 5, 2023.

Copyright © 2023 Dr. Ankita Kashyap and Prof. Krishna N. Sharma.

ISBN: 979-8223813767

Written by Dr. Ankita Kashyap and Prof. Krishna N. Sharma.

Table of Contents

DISCLAIMER

The information provided in this book is intended for general informational purposes only. The content is not meant to substitute professional medical advice, diagnosis, or treatment. Always consult with a qualified healthcare provider before making any changes to your diabetes management plan or healthcare regimen.

While every effort has been made to ensure the accuracy and completeness of the information presented, the author and publisher do not assume any responsibility for errors, omissions, or potential misinterpretations of the content. Individual responses to diabetes management strategies may vary, and what works for one person might not be suitable for another.

The book does not endorse any specific medical treatments, products, or services. Readers are encouraged to seek guidance from their healthcare providers to determine the most appropriate approaches for their unique medical conditions and needs.

Any external links or resources provided in the book are for convenience and informational purposes only. The author and publisher do not have control over the content or availability of these external sources and do not endorse or guarantee the accuracy of such information.

Readers are advised to exercise caution and use their judgment when applying the information provided in this book to their own situations. The author and publisher disclaim any liability for any direct, indirect, consequential, or other damages arising from the use of this book and its content.

By reading and using this book, readers acknowledge and accept the limitations and inherent risks associated with implementing the strategies, recommendations, and information contained herein. It is always recommended to consult a qualified healthcare professional for personalized medical advice and care.

Introduction

The Provoking Question:

Have you ever wondered why something as seemingly simple as a sore throat can leave us feeling utterly miserable? Why does it have the power to turn our lives upside down, disrupting our everyday routines and leaving us desperate for relief? Today, my dear reader, I invite you to embark on a journey of discovery as we demystify the world of strep throat.

Contextualize the Question:

In the vast landscape of medical ailments, strep throat may not be the most sinister or life-threatening. However, its ability to wield immense power over our well-being is undeniable. The soreness, the difficulty swallowing, the fever, the exhaustion—they all conspire to make even the simplest tasks feel like mountainous challenges. And yet, so often, we overlook the profound impact this seemingly minor affliction can have on our lives.

Detail the Problem:

Our understanding of strep throat is often limited to the textbook definitions and clinical descriptions that leave us grappling for answers. We find ourselves lost in a sea of confusing symptoms, ineffective remedies, and a lack of crucial information. What exactly causes this seemingly innocuous ailment to inflict such misery? Why do some individuals seem more prone to its clutches, while others seemingly escape unscathed? These are the questions that linger in the minds of countless strep throat sufferers.

Here's What Most People Do:

When faced with the torment of strep throat, we tend to rely on antiquated remedies passed down through generations. From gargling with saltwater to sipping on hot tea, we cling desperately to these age-old practices, hoping for some semblance of relief. We turn to over-the-counter medications that promise a quick fix, only to find ourselves disheartened when their effects prove fleeting. In our desperation, we seek solace in the notion that this agony is just a part of life, with no real solution in sight.

Here's the Real Solution:

But what if I told you there's a hidden world of strep throat management waiting to be revealed? A world where the conventional approaches fall by the wayside, replaced by a holistic, biopsychosocial approach that considers the multifaceted nature of our beings. In my book, "Strep Throat Demystified: Doctor's Secret Guide", I invite you to dive into this uncharted territory, where we explore the interplay between our physical health, our mental well-being, and the social factors that surround us.

By weaving together my experiences as a medical doctor and health and wellness coach, along with the expertise of my team of professionals from diverse fields, we offer a transformative perspective on strep throat management. From lifestyle modifications and dietary considerations to counseling techniques and self-help strategies, we leave no stone unturned in our quest to empower you on your journey towards recovery.

Forge a Real Connection to the Reader:

Dear reader, I know firsthand the frustration that accompanies strep throat. The helplessness as you struggle to find relief, the weariness that seeps into your bones, and the longing for answers that seem eternally out of reach. I understand the toll it takes on your body, mind, and spirit. But let me assure you, this isn't just another ailment. It's your ailment. It's your unique story, intertwined with centuries of human suffering and triumph. And it's time for you to reclaim control and rewrite the narrative of your health.

Engage Emotionally:

Close your eyes for a moment and imagine a day without the nagging pain, the relentless discomfort, and the constant uncertainty. Picture a world where strep throat no longer holds you hostage, where you can fully embrace the joys of life without the shadow of illness looming overhead. Hold onto that vision, my dear reader, for within the pages of this book lies the promise of a brighter, healthier future—one that is free from the shackles of strep throat.

Conclude with a Promise or Teaser:

So, are you ready to embark on this extraordinary journey of self-discovery and healing? Together, we will untangle the intricacies of strep throat, unlock the secrets of its origins, and unveil a comprehensive roadmap towards holistic well-being. Along the way, you will meet fellow strep throat warriors who have triumphed over adversity and uncover the tools and techniques they used to claim victory. Brace yourself, for the demystification of strep throat has only just begun. May you find solace, strength, and newfound hope within the pages that lie ahead.

Chapter 1: Understanding Strep Throat

What Is Strep Throat?

Introduction to Strep Throat:

Strep throat, a commonly experienced throat infection, is the focus of our exploration. Its prevalence is undeniable, affecting countless individuals and disrupting their daily lives. The importance of understanding this condition lies in its impact, not just physically, but also emotionally and socially. At its core, strep throat is primarily caused by a bacterial infection with Streptococcus bacteria. The reach of this infection is far-reaching, with its spread demanding our attention and understanding.

Understanding Strep Throat:

Imagine a bacterial invasion that targets the delicate tissues of the throat and tonsils, causing havoc within. This is strep throat in its essence - a bacterial infection that wreaks havoc on our throats and can leave us feeling helpless and in pain. The telltale signs of strep throat include a sore throat, fever, and swollen lymph nodes, but it doesn't stop there. Difficulty swallowing, a red, inflamed throat - these are the additional symptoms that accompany this invasive infection.

Causes of Strep Throat:

To fully comprehend strep throat, we must direct our attention to its origins. Streptococcus bacteria, specifically group A Streptococcus, serve as the primary culprits behind this infection. These pesky bacteria are transmitted through respiratory droplets, often spread by coughing, sneezing, or even talking. It is the close contact with an infected individual, such as sharing utensils or engaging in intimate activities like kissing, that heightens the risk of contracting strep throat.

How Strep Throat Differs from Other Throat Infections:

Strep throat clearly stands apart from other common throat infections, such as viral pharyngitis or tonsillitis. While these infections may also cause discomfort and pain, it is crucial to acknowledge the distinct nature of strep throat. Unlike viral infections, strep throat is specifically caused by a bacterial invasion. This distinction warrants individualized attention and treatment. Furthermore, strep throat manifests in unique ways, with the presence of white patches or pus in the throat serving as distinguishing features.

Diagnosis of Strep Throat:

Accurately diagnosing strep throat is of utmost importance in order to receive appropriate treatment. A healthcare professional, typically a doctor, is the key to unlocking this diagnosis. The process often involves a throat swab test, serving as a means to identify the presence of Streptococcus bacteria. Through this test, we gain clarity and can chart a course towards recovery.

The Impact of Strep Throat on Overall Health and Well-being:

The consequences of strep throat extend beyond the immediate discomfort and pain. If left untreated or poorly managed, strep throat can lead to severe complications. The infection may spread to other parts of the body, causing further harm and potentially resulting in conditions such as rheumatic fever or kidney problems. To prevent these potentially devastating complications, seeking medical attention and adhering to a proper treatment plan is absolutely crucial.

Conclusion:

As we conclude this exploration into the world of strep throat, we must acknowledge the multifaceted nature of this ailment. It is not simply a matter of physical discomfort, but rather a complex interplay of various factors that impact our overall health and well-being. By embracing a holistic approach, we empower ourselves on this journey towards recovery. In the following chapters, we will delve deeper into this alternative path, crafting a comprehensive roadmap that encompasses lifestyle modifications, dietary considerations, counseling techniques, and self-help strategies. Join me, dear reader, as we continue our quest to demystify strep throat and reclaim control over our health.

Signs and Symptoms

Introduction to Signs and Symptoms:

In this segment, we will explore the signs and symptoms of strep throat, a common and often misunderstood condition. Understanding these signs and symptoms is crucial for early detection and treatment, as it allows for prompt medical intervention and better management of the condition. So, let us dive into this multifaceted world and demystify the manifestations of strep throat.

The Importance of Recognizing Signs and Symptoms:

Recognizing the signs and symptoms of strep throat is of utmost importance. It enables us to take timely action and seek the necessary medical intervention. By being aware of these indicators, we can navigate through this health challenge with greater ease and ensure a speedier recovery. Prompt identification of strep throat symptoms can prevent the condition from worsening and potentially avoid complications that may arise from a delayed diagnosis.

Sore Throat:

One of the most common signs of strep throat is a sore throat. It is characterized by a sensation of discomfort and pain in the throat. This persistent irritation can make it challenging to swallow and speak, affecting daily activities. Individuals with strep throat often experience a scratchy and raw feeling in the throat, making it difficult to ignore the presence of this ailment.

Difficulty Swallowing:

Another tell-tale sign of strep throat is difficulty swallowing. The inflammation and infection caused by Streptococcus bacteria can make swallowing painful or uncomfortable. This discomfort may even lead to a loss of appetite as individuals may prefer to avoid eating or drinking due to the pain. If you find yourself struggling to swallow, it is important to consider the possibility of strep throat and seek appropriate medical care.

Fever:

Fever is a common symptom that accompanies strep throat. The body's natural response to an infection, a fever serves as an indication that something is amiss. While a fever can be caused by various factors, when combined with other signs and symptoms of strep throat, it is a strong indication that the presence of Streptococcus bacteria is causing the infection.

Swollen Tonsils:

Strep throat often presents with swollen tonsils. These two almond-shaped masses at the back of the throat may appear larger than usual, and their surface may be reddened or inflamed. In some cases, white or yellow patches may be visible on the tonsils, indicating the presence of pus. These swollen and inflamed tonsils can cause discomfort and pain, further contributing to the overall symptoms experienced by individuals with strep throat.

Other Possible Symptoms:

While sore throat, difficulty swallowing, fever, and swollen tonsils are the typical signs and symptoms of strep throat, it is important to note that these manifestations can vary from person to person. Some individuals may also experience additional symptoms such as headache, body aches, or a rash. These variations highlight the diverse ways in which strep throat can present itself and should be taken into consideration when seeking medical attention.

Seeking Medical Attention:

If you experience any of the signs and symptoms mentioned, it is essential to seek medical attention. Consulting a healthcare professional, such as a doctor, will ensure an accurate diagnosis and appropriate treatment. Through professional guidance, you can establish a tailored treatment plan and take the necessary steps towards a faster recovery.

Summary of Signs and Symptoms:

To summarize, the signs and symptoms of strep throat include a sore throat, difficulty swallowing, fever, and swollen tonsils. These indicators are the common threads that weave through the experiences of individuals with this condition. Recognizing these signs and promptly seeking medical intervention will pave the way for effective treatment and a successful journey towards reclaiming control over our health.

Diagnosis of Strep Throat:

Accurately diagnosing strep throat is crucial to receiving appropriate treatment. A healthcare professional, typically a doctor, plays a pivotal role in unlocking this diagnosis. The process often involves a throat swab test, which identifies the presence of Streptococcus bacteria. This test provides the clarity needed to chart a course towards recovery and ensure the most effective treatment plan tailored to individual needs.

The Impact of Strep Throat on Overall Health and Well-being:

The consequences of strep throat extend beyond the immediate discomfort and pain. If left untreated or poorly managed, strep throat can lead to severe complications. The infection may spread to other parts of the body, causing further harm and potentially resulting in conditions such as rheumatic fever or kidney problems. To prevent these potentially devastating complications, seeking medical attention and adhering to a proper treatment plan is absolutely crucial.

Conclusion:

As we conclude our exploration into the signs and symptoms of strep throat, we recognize the multifaceted nature of this ailment. It is not merely a matter of physical discomfort but rather a complex interplay of various factors that impact our overall health and well-being. By embracing a holistic approach, we empower ourselves on this journey towards recovery. In the following chapters, we will delve deeper into this alternative path, crafting a comprehensive roadmap that encompasses lifestyle modifications, dietary considerations, counseling techniques, and self-help strategies. Together, let us demystify strep throat and reclaim control over our health.

Diagnosing Strep Throat

Accurate diagnosis is the cornerstone of effective strep throat management, and it is essential to utilize appropriate diagnostic methods to confirm the presence of Streptococcus bacteria. In this subchapter, we will explore the different diagnostic methods used to diagnose strep throat, highlighting the importance of prompt and accurate diagnosis for appropriate treatment.

The first and most common diagnostic method for strep throat is throat swabs. This simple procedure involves a healthcare professional using a cotton swab to collect a sample from the back of the throat. It is crucial to ensure proper technique and obtain a good sample for accurate results. The swab sample is then sent to the laboratory for analysis, where it is tested for the presence of Streptococcus bacteria. Throat swabs are a reliable and widely used method of diagnosing strep throat, providing vital information for treatment decisions.

Another diagnostic method that offers a quicker turnaround time is the rapid strep test. This test can provide results within minutes, allowing for timely diagnosis and treatment. Similar to throat swabs, the procedure involves using a swab to collect a sample from the back of the throat. The swab is then inserted into a test kit that detects the presence of group A streptococcus bacteria. Rapid strep tests offer convenience and rapidity, making them a valuable tool in diagnosing strep throat, especially in urgent care settings.

Both throat swabs and rapid strep tests have been proven to be highly accurate in diagnosing strep throat. However, it is important to note that there is a slight possibility of false-negative or false-positive results. In cases where the test results are inconclusive or there is uncertainty, additional testing or clinical evaluation may be necessary to confirm the diagnosis. Healthcare professionals play a crucial role in interpreting test results correctly and prescribing appropriate treatment based on the diagnosis.

While rapid strep tests can be done at home, it is still recommended to seek medical advice and confirmation from a healthcare professional. The expertise of healthcare professionals ensures accurate diagnosis and appropriate treatment. They have the knowledge and skills to accurately interpret test results and prescribe the most effective course of treatment.

While throat swabs and rapid strep tests are the primary diagnostic methods for strep throat, there may be other less commonly used diagnostic methods in specific cases. These additional tests, such as culture tests or blood tests, may be utilized when confirmation is needed for a more severe or complicated condition. These tests help provide a comprehensive assessment of the condition, aiding in accurate diagnosis and treatment planning.

Accurate diagnosis is crucial for determining the appropriate treatment for strep throat. Prompt initiation of proper treatment can help alleviate symptoms, prevent complications, and minimize the spread of the infection. Antibiotics are the most common treatment for strep throat, and an accurate diagnosis ensures that the correct antibiotic is prescribed for effective treatment.

In conclusion, accurate diagnosis is the foundation for effective strep throat management and recovery. Throat swabs and rapid strep tests are the primary diagnostic methods used to confirm strep throat, providing valuable information to guide treatment decisions. Consulting a healthcare professional is imperative to ensure accurate diagnosis and appropriate treatment. By leveraging the expertise of healthcare professionals and utilizing proper diagnostic methods, we can demystify strep throat and take the necessary steps towards reclaiming control over our health.

Impact on Health and Well-being

The impact of untreated strep throat on a person's health and well-being cannot be underestimated. Delaying or ignoring treatment for strep throat can lead to a cascade of complications that can have long-lasting effects on the body and mind.

One of the potential complications of untreated strep throat is the development of more serious conditions, such as rheumatic fever, kidney infections, and scarlet fever. Rheumatic fever can cause inflammation in the joints, heart, and other organs, leading to long-term heart problems and joint pain. Kidney infections can result in kidney damage and chronic kidney disease. Scarlet fever can cause a rash and high fever and, if left untreated, can lead to serious complications.

But the dangers of untreated strep throat do not end there. Chronic conditions can arise from untreated strep throat, such as recurrent infections, heart problems, and joint pain. The recurrent infections can be a result of a weakened immune system as a consequence of leaving strep throat untreated. Heart problems can occur due to the spread of the strep bacteria to the heart, leading to conditions like rheumatic heart disease. Joint pain, often in the form of rheumatoid arthritis, can develop as a result of the inflammatory response triggered by untreated strep throat.

The impact on daily functioning and quality of life cannot be overlooked. The discomfort caused by untreated strep throat can make it difficult to eat, speak, and sleep. Pain and difficulty swallowing can result in loss of appetite, weight loss, and overall malnutrition. The inability to speak properly can affect personal and professional relationships. Ongoing sleep disturbances can lead to fatigue, irritability, and decreased productivity. Timely treatment is crucial to minimizing these disruptions and maintaining a good quality of life.

The emotional and psychological impact of untreated strep throat should also be acknowledged. The physical discomfort and limitations caused by strep throat can lead to feelings of frustration, anxiety, and depression. The inability to participate in activities that were once enjoyable can take a toll on mental well-being. It is important to address strep throat promptly to alleviate these emotional and psychological challenges.

Untreated strep throat can also have a significant impact on social relationships and interactions. Engaging in social activities can become difficult due to the physical discomfort and limitations caused by strep throat. Missing school or work can lead to isolation, decreased productivity, and potential strain on relationships. Addressing strep throat promptly is essential to minimize these disruptions and maintain healthy social connections.

The financial implications of leaving strep throat untreated should not be overlooked either. Prolonged illness and the need for additional medical interventions can lead to increased healthcare costs and potential loss of income. Timely treatment not only prevents potential complications but also minimizes the financial burdens associated with untreated strep throat.

Understanding the impact of untreated strep throat on health and well-being highlights the crucial importance of timely treatment. By seeking prompt medical attention, individuals can prevent potential complications, long-term effects, and preserve physical, emotional, social, and financial well-being.

To further illustrate the potential complications and long-term effects of untreated strep throat, let me share a few real-life examples and case studies. I have seen patients who, due to delayed treatment, developed rheumatic fever and had to undergo multiple surgeries to repair heart damage. I have also treated individuals who experienced recurrent infections, leading to chronic fatigue and a compromised quality of life. These cases serve as a stark reminder of the importance of learning from these examples and seeking prompt medical attention.

Now that we understand the impact of untreated strep throat, it is crucial to share this knowledge with others and raise awareness about the importance of timely treatment. By spreading awareness, we have the potential to prevent others from experiencing the negative impact of untreated strep throat. Together, we can contribute to the overall improvement of health and well-being in our communities.

In the next chapter, we will dive deeper into the different treatment options available for strep throat and how they can help alleviate symptoms, prevent complications, and promote a speedy recovery. Join me as we continue our journey to demystify strep throat and empower ourselves with knowledge and understanding.

Chapter 2: Holistic Approach to Managing Strep Throat

The Biopsychosocial Model

The Biopsychosocial Model:

When it comes to understanding and managing strep throat, it is essential to adopt a holistic approach that considers not only the biological factors but also the psychological and social elements that contribute to the condition. The biopsychosocial model provides a comprehensive framework for healthcare professionals to better understand strep throat and develop tailored treatment plans that address the individual needs of patients.

In the realm of biology, strep throat is caused by the Streptococcus bacteria. These bacteria invade the throat, leading to symptoms such as sore throat, fever, and difficulty swallowing. Understanding the biological factors at play is crucial in determining the appropriate course of treatment. For instance, the severity of the infection and the length of recovery can vary depending on the immune response of the individual. By recognizing the biological factors, healthcare professionals can better tailor their treatment recommendations, including the use of antibiotics and supportive measures to boost the immune system.

However, it is equally important to consider the psychological factors that can influence strep throat. Stress, anxiety, and other emotional factors have been shown to weaken the immune system, making individuals more susceptible to infections. With strep throat being a recurring condition for some individuals, the psychological impact of living with this chronic illness cannot be overlooked. It is imperative to address the emotional well-being of patients, offering support and counseling to help them cope with the challenges of managing their condition.

The social factors also play a significant role in strep throat management. Living conditions, socioeconomic status, and access to healthcare can all influence an individual's risk of developing strep throat and their ability to effectively manage the condition. For instance, individuals living in crowded or unhygienic conditions are more likely to contract the strep bacteria. Additionally, individuals lacking access to healthcare facilities may face delays in diagnosis and treatment, prolonging their recovery time. By understanding the social factors at play, healthcare professionals can provide targeted interventions that address these barriers and improve overall outcomes.

Integrating the biopsychosocial model in strep throat management allows healthcare professionals to develop comprehensive treatment plans that address all aspects of a patient's well-being. By considering the biological, psychological, and social factors, healthcare professionals can provide holistic and personalized care that goes beyond simply prescribing antibiotics. This approach not only improves patient outcomes but also supports overall well-being and quality of life.

Applying the biopsychosocial model to strep throat management involves several strategies. Healthcare professionals may recommend lifestyle modifications such as adequate rest and hydration, a healthy diet, and regular exercise to support the body's immune system. Stress-management techniques such as relaxation exercises, mindfulness, and counseling can help individuals cope with the emotional challenges of managing a chronic illness. Additionally, healthcare professionals may connect patients with support groups or community resources to address social factors and provide a network of understanding and encouragement.

The benefits of adopting the biopsychosocial model in strep throat management are significant. By taking a comprehensive approach, healthcare professionals can provide individualized care that addresses each patient's unique needs. This model encourages communication and collaboration between healthcare professionals and patients, leading to a stronger therapeutic alliance. By considering all factors that contribute to the condition, healthcare professionals aim to improve treatment outcomes, reduce the recurrence of strep throat, and enhance overall well-being.

In conclusion, the biopsychosocial model is a valuable framework that aids in understanding and managing strep throat. By incorporating biological, psychological, and social factors into the treatment plan, healthcare professionals can provide holistic care that addresses the diverse needs of each patient. It is essential for patients to recognize the importance of these factors and actively participate in their own treatment and wellness journey. By considering all aspects of health, individuals can improve their overall physical and mental well-being, leading to a more fulfilling and healthier life.

Lifestyle Modifications

Introduction to Lifestyle Modifications for Strep Throat Management:

As I reflect on my years of medical practice and my passion for holistic healthcare and wellness, I am continuously reminded of the immense impact that lifestyle modifications can have on a person's health. Strep throat, a common and often uncomfortable infection, is no exception to this rule. Lifestyle factors can play a significant role in determining the severity and duration of strep throat symptoms. By making targeted lifestyle changes, individuals can not only alleviate their immediate discomfort but also support their body's natural healing process. In this chapter, we will delve deep into the specific lifestyle modifications that can aid in the management of strep throat, providing a comprehensive guide to promote optimal recovery and overall well-being.

The Power of Proper Rest:

When it comes to strep throat management, few things are as crucial as proper rest. Sleep is a restorative process that allows our bodies to redirect energy towards fighting off the infection. Inadequate rest can weaken the immune system, delay recovery, and worsen symptoms. To ensure optimal rest, it is essential to create a conducive sleep environment. This includes implementing factors such as a cool, dark, and quiet room, comfortable bedding, and a consistent sleep routine. By prioritizing rest and establishing healthy sleep habits, individuals can support their body's healing process and find relief from the discomfort of strep throat.

Hydration: The Key to Soothing a Sore Throat:

A sore throat is one of the most uncomfortable symptoms of strep throat. Proper hydration can play a significant role in soothing the irritation and discomfort caused by this symptom. Drinking plenty of fluids helps keep the throat moist, provides relief, and aids in the healing process. It is important to choose the right beverages to maximize hydration and ease symptoms. Herbal teas, lukewarm soups, and fruit-infused water can all be excellent choices. Additionally, incorporating hydration into daily routines can be enhanced with creative ideas such as homemade popsicles, ice chips, and herbal throat sprays. By prioritizing hydration, individuals can find relief from the discomfort of strep throat and expedite their recovery.

The Art of Avoiding Irritants:

During the management of strep throat, it is crucial to avoid irritants that can worsen symptoms. Irritants can further inflame the throat, exacerbating discomfort and prolonging the healing process. Common irritants include smoking, exposure to harsh chemicals, pollution, and excessive talking or shouting. It is essential to minimize exposure to these irritants by using air purifiers, avoiding crowded and polluted areas, and wearing a mask when necessary. By diligently avoiding irritants, individuals can create an environment that supports the healing process and minimizes the impact of strep throat symptoms.

Creating a Restorative Environment:

The physical environment in which individuals recover from strep throat can significantly impact their symptoms and well-being. Creating a clean and dust-free environment is crucial. Dust can exacerbate respiratory symptoms, worsening the discomfort of strep throat. Regular cleaning routines, the use of air purifiers, and dust-free bedding and furnishings can significantly reduce the presence of allergens and promote faster healing. Additionally, incorporating the use of humidifiers and essential oils can further soothe throat discomfort and promote relaxation during the recovery process. By creating a restorative environment, individuals can enhance their recovery from strep throat and alleviate their symptoms.

The Role of Nutrition in Strep Throat Management:

Proper nutrition plays a vital role in supporting the immune system during strep throat recovery. A balanced and nutritious diet helps supply the body with the essential nutrients it needs to fight off the infection. However, considering the throat's sensitivity, it is crucial to choose foods that are easy to swallow and gentle on the throat. Soft, warm foods such as soups, smoothies, and mashed vegetables are excellent choices. Additionally, incorporating nutrient-dense meals and snacks can aid in the healing process. Foods rich in vitamin C, zinc, and antioxidants can support overall immune function and expedite recovery. By prioritizing a healthy diet, individuals can nourish their bodies and promote optimal healing during their strep throat management journey.

The Power of Gentle Exercise:

While it may seem counterintuitive to engage in physical activity during strep throat recovery, gentle exercise can play a significant role in supporting the healing process. Light, low-impact exercises such as walking, stretching, and gentle yoga can improve circulation, boost the immune system, and promote overall well-being. Exercise helps stimulate the lymphatic system, which aids in the removal of toxins and waste products from the body. However, it is crucial to listen to the body's signals and engage in exercise only when it feels comfortable and manageable. By incorporating gentle exercise into the strep throat management plan, individuals can support their body's healing process and enhance their overall well-being.

Managing Stress and Anxiety:

Stress and anxiety can significantly impact the body's immune system and worsen strep throat symptoms. The emotional challenges that accompany the management of a chronic illness cannot be overlooked. Incorporating stress-management techniques into daily routines is essential for individuals with strep throat. Deep breathing exercises, meditation, relaxation techniques, and counseling can all be effective tools in managing stress and anxiety. Additionally, cultivating mindfulness and being present in each moment can help individuals navigate the ups and downs of the strep throat management journey.

By prioritizing emotional well-being, individuals can support their immune system and improve symptom management.

Social Support for Strengthening Resilience:

The strep throat management journey can be challenging, both physically and emotionally. Social support plays a crucial role in strengthening resilience and improving outcomes. Connecting with loved ones, joining support groups, and engaging in open and honest communication can provide individuals with the understanding and encouragement they need. In today's digital age, even during physical distancing, social connections can still be fostered through virtual platforms and online communities. By actively seeking and nurturing social support, individuals can find solace in shared experiences and enhance their strep throat management journey.

Developing Healthy Habits for Long-Term Prevention:

While managing the immediate symptoms of strep throat is essential, it is equally important to develop healthy habits for long-term prevention. Good oral hygiene practices, such as regular brushing and flossing, can help prevent the recurrence of strep throat and other oral infections. Staying adequately hydrated, managing stress through healthy coping mechanisms, and maintaining a balanced diet rich in immune-boosting nutrients are all crucial in preventing future episodes. Regular medical check-ups and immunizations are also vital in identifying potential risks and taking proactive measures to maintain optimal health. By adopting these healthy habits, individuals can reduce the likelihood of future strep throat infections and promote long-term well-being.

Conclusion - Encouraging a Holistic Lifestyle:

As we conclude this chapter on lifestyle modifications for strep throat management, it is evident that a holistic approach is essential in promoting optimal recovery and overall well-being. By prioritizing rest, hydration, and avoiding irritants, individuals can create an environment that supports the healing process. Proper nutrition, gentle exercise, stress management, and social support all contribute to improved outcomes and overall wellness. It is crucial for individuals to recognize the importance of these lifestyle modifications and actively incorporate them into their daily routines. By embracing a holistic lifestyle, individuals can not only manage strep throat effectively but also enhance their overall physical and mental well-being, leading to a more fulfilling and healthier life.

With this foundation of lifestyle modifications in place, the next chapter will delve into complementary and alternative therapies, offering a comprehensive guide to further support strep throat management and recovery.

Nutrition and Diet Planning

Nutrition and diet planning are crucial components in supporting the immune system and promoting recovery from strep throat. A healthy diet provides essential nutrients and vitamins necessary for immune function, helping the body to fight off infections and expedite the healing process.

The immune system plays a vital role in defending the body against infections like strep throat. A strong immune system can help in faster recovery by effectively attacking and eliminating the pathogens causing the infection. Therefore, it is essential to support the immune system through proper nutrition.

Specific nutrients have been found to be beneficial for immune function. These include vitamin C, which is known for its immune-stimulating properties and can be obtained from sources such as citrus fruits, strawberries, and bell peppers. Vitamin D, which can be obtained from sunlight exposure and certain foods like fatty fish and fortified dairy products, also plays a crucial role in supporting immune function. Zinc, found in foods like lean meats, seafood, and legumes, is another nutrient that supports immune function and aids in recovery. Lastly, antioxidants, found in fruits, vegetables, and whole grains, help protect the immune system from damage caused by free radicals and support overall immune health.

A balanced diet is essential in providing all the necessary nutrients for optimal immune function. A well-rounded meal plan should include a variety of fruits, vegetables, whole grains, lean proteins, and healthy fats. For example, a typical day's meal plan may consist of a breakfast smoothie containing spinach, berries, and almond butter; a lunch consisting of grilled chicken breast, quinoa, and steamed vegetables; and a dinner of salmon, brown rice, and sautéed greens. Snacks can include nuts, seeds, and fresh fruits.

Hydration also plays a role in supporting the immune system. Drinking enough water helps flush out toxins from the body and maintain proper bodily functions. It is recommended to consume at least 8 glasses of water per day. Additionally, herbal teas, lukewarm soups, and fruit-infused water can be excellent choices to enhance hydration. Creative ideas such as homemade popsicles, ice chips, and herbal throat sprays can also help prioritize hydration and alleviate the discomfort of strep throat.

While focusing on a healthy diet, it is equally important to avoid inflammatory foods that can weaken the immune system. Processed foods, sugary snacks, and excessive alcohol consumption should be minimized or avoided. These foods can cause inflammation in the body and impair immune function, thus hindering the recovery process.

Maintaining a healthy gut is also crucial for a strong immune system. The gut microbiota plays a significant role in the immune response. Including probiotic-rich foods like yogurt, kefir, sauerkraut, and kimchi in the diet can help support a healthy gut microbiota and strengthen the immune system.

Maintaining a healthy weight is another important aspect of supporting the immune system during strep throat recovery. Obesity has been associated with impaired immune function, making it harder for the body to fight off infections and prolonging the recovery process. By adopting a balanced diet and engaging in regular exercise, individuals can support their immune system and optimize their overall health.

Meal timing and regular eating patterns also play a role in promoting optimal immune function. Skipping meals or following restrictive diets can negatively impact the immune system. It is important to listen to the body's hunger and fullness cues and provide it with consistent nourishment throughout the day.

Practical tips for meal planning and preparation can be helpful in implementing a healthy diet. It is recommended to plan meals ahead of time, choose immune-boosting recipes, and incorporate a variety of nutrient-rich foods into daily meals. Adding herbs and spices like turmeric, ginger, garlic, and oregano to meals can also provide additional immune-boosting benefits.

While nutrition from whole foods should be the primary focus, supplements may be considered in certain cases to support the immune system. It is important to consult with a healthcare professional before starting any supplementation regimen to ensure appropriate dosage and safety.

Individuals with specific dietary restrictions or allergies should be mindful of alternative options to meet their nutritional needs. There are numerous resources available, including substitutes for common allergens and specialized diets like vegetarian, vegan, or gluten-free.

Lastly, it is important to remember the importance of ongoing dietary choices and maintaining a healthy lifestyle even after recovering from strep throat. Nutrition plays a significant role in overall health and well-being, and making informed dietary choices is crucial for long-term wellness.

In summary, nutrition and diet planning are essential in supporting the immune system and promoting recovery from strep throat. A balanced diet, rich in immune-boosting nutrients, hydration, avoiding inflammatory foods, maintaining a healthy gut, and a healthy weight are all crucial components of a comprehensive nutrition plan. By incorporating these principles into daily life, individuals can optimize their immune function, expedite their recovery from strep throat, and enhance their overall well-being.

Coping Strategies and Stress Management

Coping Strategies and Stress Management:

Living with strep throat can be physically and emotionally challenging. In addition to addressing the physical symptoms, it is important to recognize and manage the stress that can accompany the condition. Coping strategies and stress management techniques are essential tools in navigating the recovery journey. By embracing these strategies, strep throat patients can promote a faster recovery, alleviate symptoms, and improve their overall well-being.

The physical impact of strep throat on stress levels cannot be understated. The discomfort and pain associated with the condition can cause increased stress and anxiety. Swallowing becomes a painful experience, sleep may be disrupted, and an overall feeling of lethargy can set in. These physical challenges can exacerbate stress levels, further hindering the recovery process.

Incorporating stress reduction techniques into daily life is a critical component of managing strep throat. Mindfulness techniques such as deep breathing exercises and guided meditation can help individuals find calm and relax their body and mind. By practicing these techniques regularly, patients can better manage their stress levels and improve their overall well-being.

The connection between stress and the immune system is a vital aspect to consider when managing strep throat. Chronic stress can weaken the immune system, making symptoms more severe and prolonging the recovery process. It is crucial to find healthy and effective ways to manage stress in order to support the immune system and aid in faster recovery.

Exercise can play a significant role in stress management for strep throat patients. While vigorous exercise may not be appropriate during the acute phase of the illness, gentle stretching or low-impact activities can help reduce stress levels. Physical activity releases endorphins, which are known as "feel-good" hormones, helping to alleviate stress and improve overall well-being.

Nurturing emotional well-being while living with strep throat is equally important. Journaling, practicing gratitude, and seeking emotional support from loved ones or support groups can provide an outlet for emotions related to the condition. By acknowledging and processing these emotions, individuals can better cope with the challenges of strep throat and promote their emotional well-being.

Creating a supportive environment is crucial for stress reduction. Decluttering physical space, establishing boundaries, and surrounding oneself with positive influences can greatly contribute to stress management. By optimizing their surroundings, individuals can create a peaceful atmosphere that promotes relaxation and reduces stress.

Mind-body techniques offer a powerful way to cope with strep throat. Guided imagery, progressive muscle relaxation, and biofeedback are techniques that can provide relief from pain and promote relaxation. By integrating these techniques into their daily routine, individuals can regain a sense of control over their condition and find comfort during the recovery process.

Relaxation techniques are also valuable tools for stress reduction. Aromatherapy, warm baths with essential oils, and soothing music can create a calming atmosphere and help individuals unwind. Exploring different relaxation techniques and finding what resonates with them can support stress management and overall well-being.

While self-help techniques are valuable, seeking professional help for stress management should not be overlooked. Therapists, psychologists, and counselors can provide additional support and guidance during the strep throat journey. Their expertise can help individuals develop personalized coping strategies and promote emotional well-being.

It is important to integrate coping strategies into the overall treatment plan for strep throat. By addressing both the physical and emotional aspects of the condition, a holistic approach can enhance the effectiveness of medical interventions. Communication with the healthcare team is crucial, as they can provide guidance and support in developing coping strategies that align with individual needs.

In conclusion, coping strategies and stress management techniques are essential tools in the strep throat recovery process. By actively implementing these strategies, individuals can alleviate stress, improve symptom management, and enhance their overall well-being. It is important to persevere and explore various coping strategies to find what works best for each individual. With a comprehensive approach to stress management, strep throat patients can effectively navigate their journey towards holistic wellness.

Chapter 3: Self-Care Techniques for Strep Throat Patients

Natural Remedies for Symptom Relief

Introduction to Natural Remedies for Symptom Relief

In this subchapter, I will delve into the world of natural remedies, exploring their unique benefits in alleviating the symptoms of strep throat. While conventional medications can provide relief, incorporating natural remedies into your treatment plan can enhance your body's healing process and restore your well-being. Through the use of herbal teas, gargling with saltwater, and throat lozenges, you can find solace from the discomfort caused by strep throat and aid in your recovery.

Herbal Teas for Symptom Relief

Herbal teas have long been revered for their therapeutic properties, and they are particularly effective in soothing the symptoms of strep throat. Lavender tea, famous for its calming and aromatic nature, not only helps alleviate throat pain but also aids in relaxing the body and promoting restful sleep. Chamomile tea, with its anti-inflammatory effects, works wonders in reducing the swelling and soreness in your throat, allowing you to find relief from the incessant discomfort. Echinacea tea, known for its immune-boosting properties, can help bolster your body's defenses and speed up your recovery process. To prepare these teas, steep a teaspoon of dried herbs or a tea bag in hot water for about 10 minutes. Add a touch of honey to enhance the taste if desired, and sip on these concoctions throughout the day to maximize the effectiveness.

Gargling with Saltwater for Symptom Relief

Gargling with saltwater has been a trusted remedy for throat ailments since ancient times, and for good reason. The gentle saline solution acts as an anti-inflammatory agent, reducing the swelling in your throat and providing instant relief. To prepare the saltwater solution, simply dissolve half a teaspoon of salt in warm water until it completely dissolves. Gently gargle with the solution for 30 seconds, allowing the mixture to coat your throat. Repeat this process multiple times a day to experience the soothing and healing effects of saltwater gargling.

Using Throat Lozenges for Symptom Relief

Throat lozenges serve as a natural remedy for strep throat symptoms, targeting specific discomforts such as sore throat and cough. Made with a combination of herbs and soothing ingredients, these lozenges work to numb the pain, reduce inflammation, and provide a protective coating for the throat. Honey lemon lozenges, for example, incorporate the antibacterial properties of honey and the vitamin C-rich tanginess of lemon, offering both relief and immune support. Menthol-based lozenges can provide a cooling sensation, relieving irritation and promoting easier swallowing. Choose the lozenges that suit your symptoms and preferences, and allow them to dissolve slowly in your mouth, ensuring that their healing properties are dispersed evenly.

Additional Natural Remedies for Symptom Relief

Beyond herbal teas, saltwater gargling, and throat lozenges, there are a multitude of natural remedies that can provide further relief from strep throat symptoms. The combination of honey and lemon, a classic remedy, can be mixed together to create a soothing elixir that helps relieve pain and promotes healing. Drinking ginger tea, with its anti-inflammatory and warming properties, can ease throat discomfort and aid in digestion. Steam inhalation, achieved by leaning over a bowl of hot water and inhaling the steam, can provide immediate relief from congestion and help clear your airways. Embrace these additional remedies with caution and tailor them to your specific needs, always taking into consideration any allergies or sensitivities you may have.

Safety Precautions and Considerations

As with any form of treatment, it is important to exercise a degree of caution when using natural remedies for strep throat. While generally safe, some individuals may have allergies or sensitivities to certain herbs or ingredients. It is crucial to consult with a healthcare professional before incorporating any new remedies into your treatment plan, especially if you have any underlying health conditions or are taking other medications. Always follow the instructions for preparation and consumption carefully, and discontinue use if you experience any adverse reactions or if your symptoms worsen.

Personal Stories of Success with Natural Remedies

Throughout my years as a healthcare professional and health and wellness coach, I have had the privilege of witnessing numerous success stories of individuals finding relief through natural remedies for strep throat. One particular patient, Sarah, had been suffering from severe throat pain and difficulty swallowing. Through the use of herbal teas and throat lozenges, she was able to find immense relief within a few days. Another patient, James, embraced the practice of saltwater gargling and saw a significant reduction in throat inflammation, allowing him to sleep through the night. These personal stories serve as a testament to the power and effectiveness of natural remedies, inspiring us all to explore alternative solutions in our journey towards symptom relief and well-being.

As you embark on your own path towards alleviating the symptoms of strep throat, consider the natural remedies presented in this subchapter. By embracing holistic healthcare practices and incorporating lifestyle modifications, you can empower yourself to take charge of your health and well-being. Remember, however, that although these remedies can provide significant relief, it is essential to consult with a healthcare professional to ensure safe and effective treatment. Through the incorporation of natural remedies and the guidance of health and wellness experts, you can uncover the secrets to demystifying strep throat and restore yourself to optimal health.

Effective Home Remedies

Introduction to Effective Home Remedies

In this segment, I would like to share with you a variety of effective home remedies that can provide relief from strep throat symptoms. These remedies are natural, easily accessible, and can be used alongside conventional medical treatments to enhance relief. By incorporating these remedies into your daily routine, you can experience soothing and healing effects that will help you on your journey towards wellness.

The Importance of Home Remedies

Home remedies have long been used as an alternative approach to healthcare. They offer a multitude of benefits, including being inexpensive, easily accessible, and often free from harmful side effects. Home remedies can provide relief from strep throat symptoms and help enhance the body's natural healing process. When used in conjunction with conventional treatments, they can accelerate recovery and improve overall well-being.

Steam Inhalation

One effective home remedy for strep throat is steam inhalation. By inhaling steam, you can provide relief to your throat, reduce inflammation, and promote healing. To perform steam inhalation, bring a pot of water to a boil and carefully inhale the steam by leaning over the pot, making sure to cover your head with a towel to trap the steam. Take slow, deep breaths for about 10-15 minutes, allowing the steam to penetrate your airways and provide soothing relief.

Warm Compresses

Another home remedy that can help ease strep throat pain is the use of warm compresses. Applying a warm compress to your throat can help reduce swelling, alleviate pain, and promote comfort. To make a warm compress, soak a clean cloth in warm water, wring out any excess moisture, and place it over your throat. Leave it on for about 10-15 minutes, allowing the warmth to penetrate deep into the tissues. Repeat this process several times a day to experience the full benefits of this soothing remedy.

Herbal Teas

Herbal teas can be a soothing and comforting home remedy for strep throat. Specific herbs, such as chamomile or ginger, can provide relief from symptoms and promote healing. Chamomile tea has anti-inflammatory properties that can help soothe the throat, while ginger tea has warming and anti-inflammatory effects that can aid in digestion and ease discomfort. To prepare herbal teas, steep the desired herbs in hot water for about 10 minutes, strain, and drink while still warm. Sipping on these calming teas throughout the day can provide relief and comfort.

Gargling with Salt Water

Gargling with salt water is a time-tested home remedy for strep throat. Salt water can help reduce inflammation, kill bacteria, and relieve discomfort. To gargle with salt water, dissolve half a teaspoon of salt in a cup of warm water and mix thoroughly. Take a sip of the mixture and tilt your head back, allowing the liquid to reach the back of your throat. Gargle for about 30 seconds, making sure to focus on the areas that are most painful. Repeat this process multiple times a day to experience the soothing and healing effects of saltwater gargling.

Honey and Lemon Remedies

Honey and lemon are powerhouse ingredients that can provide immense relief for strep throat symptoms. Honey has natural antibacterial properties and can soothe the throat, while lemon provides a boost of vitamin C to support the immune system. Combining the two can create powerful remedies that address both the symptoms and the underlying infection. One popular remedy is honey-lemon water, where you mix a teaspoon of honey and the juice of half a lemon in a cup of warm water and drink it slowly. Another option is honey-lemon ginger tea, where you add grated ginger to the mixture for added anti-inflammatory effects. Sip on these remedies several times a day for maximum relief and immune support.

Eucalyptus Oil Inhalation

Inhalation of eucalyptus oil can be an effective home remedy for strep throat. Eucalyptus oil has antimicrobial properties and can help relieve congestion. To inhale eucalyptus oil, add a few drops to a bowl of hot water, carefully lean over the bowl, and cover your head with a towel. Breathe deeply to allow the steam and aroma of the oil to penetrate your airways. This can provide immediate relief from congestion and help clear your airways.

Aloe Vera Gel

Aloe vera gel is a natural remedy that can help reduce inflammation, soothe the throat, and promote healing in cases of strep throat. To use aloe vera gel, apply a small amount directly to the throat and gently massage it in. Allow the gel to sit on the throat for a few minutes before swallowing. The cooling and soothing properties of aloe vera gel can provide relief and comfort.

Conclusion

In conclusion, there are a variety of effective home remedies that can provide relief from strep throat symptoms. By incorporating these natural remedies into your treatment plan, you can enhance the healing process and alleviate discomfort. Remember to consult with a healthcare professional before trying any new remedies, especially if you have underlying health conditions or are taking other medications. With the proper guidance and the use of these holistic remedies, you can demystify strep throat and restore yourself to optimal health.

Importance of Hygiene Practices

Introduction to the subchapter:

Maintaining proper hygiene practices is crucial in preventing the spread of strep throat and promoting faster recovery. In this subchapter, we will explore the various hygiene practices that play a vital role in safeguarding against this infection. By incorporating these practices into our daily lives, we can reduce the risk of transmission and create a healthier environment for ourselves and those around us.

Hand hygiene:

One of the most fundamental hygiene practices in preventing the transmission of strep throat is regular handwashing. Our hands come into contact with numerous surfaces throughout the day, many of which can harbor bacteria. Proper handwashing technique involves using warm water and soap, rubbing the hands together for at least 20 seconds, including the backs of the hands, fingertips, and under the nails. It is important to wash hands before meals, after using the restroom, and after coughing or sneezing. In situations where handwashing is not possible, such as when traveling, hand sanitizers with at least 60% alcohol can be used to effectively kill bacteria.

Respiratory hygiene:

Respiratory hygiene plays a significant role in preventing the spread of strep throat. When we cough or sneeze, tiny droplets containing infectious bacteria are released into the air. To minimize the risk of transmission, it is essential to cover the mouth and nose with a tissue or the elbow. Using tissues helps in capturing the droplets, and promptly disposing of them in a closed bin prevents contamination. If a tissue is not available, using the elbow as a cover can also prevent the dispersal of infectious particles.

Surface hygiene:

Regularly cleaning and disinfecting commonly touched surfaces is essential in preventing the spread of strep throat. Surfaces such as doorknobs, light switches, and countertops can become contaminated with bacteria and serve as a source of transmission. Disinfectants that are effective against strep throat bacteria should be used to clean these surfaces thoroughly. By establishing a routine of regular surface cleaning, we can minimize the risk of cross-contamination and create a safe environment.

Personal hygiene:

Maintaining good personal hygiene is crucial in preventing the spread and recurrence of strep throat. Bathing or showering regularly helps remove bacteria from the body, reducing the chances of infection. It is essential to avoid sharing personal items such as towels, toothbrushes, or utensils, as these can easily transmit bacteria from one person to another. By prioritizing personal hygiene, we can reduce the risk of reinfection and create a healthier lifestyle.

Food hygiene:

Practicing good food hygiene is imperative in preventing strep throat. Properly handling, cooking, and storing food helps avoid contamination. Hands should be washed thoroughly before preparing or handling food, and raw and cooked foods should be kept separate to prevent cross-contamination. Cooking food to the appropriate temperature ensures that any bacteria present are destroyed. By practicing food hygiene, we can safeguard against strep throat and maintain overall health.

Clothing and laundry hygiene:

Clothing and laundry hygiene also play a role in preventing the spread of strep throat. Regularly washing clothes, particularly those that come into contact with the mouth and nose, helps eliminate bacteria. Beddings should also be washed frequently to maintain a clean sleeping environment. It is important to avoid sharing clothes and personal items with others, as this can lead to the transmission of bacteria and potential infection.

Hygiene in public places:

Practicing good hygiene in public places is crucial in preventing the transmission of strep throat. Using clean public facilities and properly disposing of waste helps reduce the risk of contamination. It is important to maintain personal hygiene practices even outside of our homes to create a safe and hygienic environment for ourselves and others.

Hygiene practices in healthcare settings:

Strict hygiene practices in healthcare settings are essential to prevent the spread of strep throat. Healthcare professionals adhere to personal protective equipment requirements and maintain proper sanitation protocols to ensure patient safety. By prioritizing hygiene in healthcare settings, we can reduce the risk of nosocomial infections and create a safer environment for patients and healthcare providers.

Conclusion and summary:

In summary, hygiene practices are vital in preventing the spread of strep throat and promoting faster recovery. By incorporating hand hygiene, respiratory hygiene, surface hygiene, personal hygiene, food hygiene, clothing and laundry hygiene, hygiene in public places, and hygiene practices in healthcare settings into our daily routines, we can reduce the risk of transmission and create a healthier environment. These practices not only help in preventing strep throat but also contribute to overall health and well-being. By demystifying strep throat and emphasizing the importance of hygiene practices, we can empower individuals to take charge of their health and prevent the spread of this infection.

Transition to the next subchapter or chapter:

With a thorough understanding of hygiene practices, we can now delve into the next subchapter, where we will explore the role of nutrition in strep throat prevention and recovery. By adopting a holistic approach to healthcare and combining proper hygiene practices with a nutritious diet, we can optimize our immune system and promote overall wellness.

Rest and Relaxation Techniques

Introduction to Rest and Relaxation Techniques:

In the journey towards healing from strep throat, rest and relaxation techniques play a crucial role in supporting the body's natural recovery process. As a medical doctor and health and wellness coach, I have witnessed the transformative power of these techniques in improving overall well-being. In this segment, we will explore various rest and relaxation techniques that can be incorporated into daily routines to promote relaxation, reduce stress, and aid in the healing process. From meditation to yoga, deep breathing exercises to guided imagery, and aromatherapy to mindfulness practices, we will delve deep into the realm of self-care and self-healing.

The Power of Meditation:

Meditation, a practice that has been embraced for centuries, holds immense potential in alleviating the symptoms and promoting the healing process for those with strep throat. By redirecting our attention inward and embracing a state of mindfulness, we can effectively reduce the stress that often accompanies illness. Research has shown that meditation has the ability to lower cortisol levels, the hormone responsible for stress, allowing the body to activate its own healing mechanisms. Additionally, regular meditation practice has been shown to improve sleep quality, which is crucial for the body's restoration and recovery.

There are various meditation techniques that strep throat patients can explore. One such technique is mindfulness meditation, where one focuses on the present moment, observing their thoughts and sensations without judgment. Another technique is loving-kindness meditation, where one cultivates a sense of compassion and love towards themselves and others. By incorporating meditation into their daily routine, strep throat patients can tap into their own inner reservoir of resilience and well-being.

Deep Breathing Exercises for Relaxation:

Deep breathing exercises are an accessible and effective way to promote relaxation and relieve stress. By consciously focusing on our breath and engaging in slow, deep breaths, we can activate the body's relaxation response. This response triggers a decrease in heart rate, blood pressure, and muscle tension, creating a state of calm within the body.

One simple deep breathing technique that strep throat patients can practice is diaphragmatic breathing. This involves taking slow, deep breaths, allowing the diaphragm to expand fully. Another technique is alternate nostril breathing, where one closes off one nostril with the thumb and inhales deeply through the other, then switches nostrils and exhales through the opposite nostril. These exercises can be practiced anywhere, at any time, providing an immediate sense of relaxation and relief from the symptoms of strep throat.

Progressive Muscle Relaxation for Physical and Mental Relaxation:

Progressive muscle relaxation is a technique that activates both physical and mental relaxation. By systematically tensing and releasing different muscle groups in the body, we can release tension and promote a deep sense of relaxation. This technique involves consciously tensing a specific muscle group for a few seconds, then releasing the tension and allowing the muscle to relax fully.

Strep throat patients can engage in progressive muscle relaxation by starting from the toes and working their way up towards the head, tensing and relaxing each muscle group along the way. This can be done while lying down or sitting in a comfortable position. Regular practice of this technique not only promotes relaxation but also enhances body awareness, allowing individuals to identify and release physical tension that may be exacerbating their symptoms.

Guided Imagery for Relaxation and Healing:

Guided imagery harnesses the power of visualization to create a sense of calm and support the body's healing process. By engaging the senses and imagining peaceful and healing scenes, strep throat patients can tap into their own inner healing potential. Guided imagery can be practiced using scripts or audio recordings, allowing individuals to follow along and immerse themselves in a deeply relaxing and healing experience.

During guided imagery, patients can close their eyes and imagine themselves in a serene location, such as a beach or a forest. They can visualize the gentle sound of waves, the warmth of the sun on their skin, or the scent of fresh flowers. By immersing themselves in these positive and calming images, strep throat patients can counteract the stress and discomfort associated with their illness, promoting a more peaceful and healing state of being.

Aromatherapy for Relaxation and Mood Enhancement:

Aromatherapy, the use of essential oils for therapeutic purposes, offers a natural and holistic way to promote relaxation and enhance mood. Certain essential oils, such as lavender, chamomile, and eucalyptus, have been shown to possess calming and soothing properties.

Strep throat patients can incorporate aromatherapy into their daily routines by using essential oil diffusers, adding a few drops of essential oil to a warm bath, or creating homemade sprays to freshen their living spaces. The gentle scent and therapeutic properties of these oils can create a serene and inviting environment, promoting relaxation and supporting the healing process.

Yoga and Stretching for Mind-Body Connection:

Yoga, an ancient practice that combines physical postures, breathing exercises, and meditation, offers a multitude of benefits for strep throat patients. This practice not only enhances flexibility and strength but also establishes a harmonious mind-body connection. By moving through different yoga postures, individuals can release physical tension, reduce muscle stiffness, and improve overall circulation. Additionally, the focus on breath and mindfulness cultivates a sense of inner calm and relaxation.

For strep throat patients, beginner-friendly yoga poses can be incorporated into their daily routines. Simple stretches, such as neck rolls, shoulder rolls, and gentle twists, can alleviate tension in the neck and upper body, which are common areas of discomfort for those with strep throat. Engaging in a regular yoga practice not only supports physical healing but also nourishes the mind and promotes overall well-being.

Mindfulness Practices for Present-Moment Awareness:

Mindfulness, the practice of being fully present in the current moment, offers strep throat patients a powerful tool for relaxation and stress reduction. By cultivating awareness of our thoughts, sensations, and emotions without judgment, we can create a sense of calm and tranquility within ourselves. Mindfulness can be practiced in various daily activities, such as eating, walking, or even brushing our teeth.

To incorporate mindfulness into their healing journey, strep throat patients can start by dedicating a few minutes each day to practicing mindful breathing. By tuning into the sensations of the breath, they can anchor themselves in the present moment and experience a sense of lightness and ease. As they progress in their mindfulness practice, they can begin to expand their awareness to other aspects of their daily lives, allowing them to fully immerse themselves in the present moment and find respite from the challenges of their illness.

Other Rest and Relaxation Techniques:

In addition to the specific techniques discussed above, strep throat patients can explore other rest and relaxation techniques based on their individual preferences and needs. Acupuncture, an ancient Chinese healing modality, has been shown to promote relaxation and alleviate pain. Massage therapy offers a hands-on approach to releasing tension and promoting overall well-being. Music therapy, through soothing melodies and rhythm, can induce a deep sense of relaxation and emotional healing.

It is crucial for patients to consult with healthcare professionals or experts in these fields to determine the best approach for their unique circumstances. By exploring these additional rest and relaxation techniques, strep throat patients can tap into a wellspring of practices aimed at supporting their healing journey.

Conclusion and Encouragement to Explore Rest and Relaxation Techniques:

In conclusion, rest and relaxation techniques are potent tools that can aid in the healing process and promote overall well-being for those with strep throat. By integrating various techniques, such as meditation, deep breathing exercises, progressive muscle relaxation, guided imagery, aromatherapy, yoga, and mindfulness practices, individuals can create a self-care routine that supports their physical and mental health. I encourage strep throat patients to explore these techniques with an open mind and a willingness to prioritize their rest and relaxation. As they embark on this journey, they will discover the profound impact that rest and relaxation can have on their healing process, empowering them to take an active role in their own well-being. Remember, the journey towards healing is a personal one, and by embracing rest and relaxation, strep throat patients can create a sacred space within themselves for wholeness and restoration.

Chapter 4: Complementary and Alternative Therapies

Acupuncture and Acupressure

As a medical doctor and health and wellness coach, I always strive to provide my patients with a comprehensive approach to healing and wellbeing. In my practice, I have witnessed the transformative power of acupuncture and acupressure in promoting balance and restoring the body's natural healing abilities. These ancient Chinese modalities have been used for centuries to address a wide range of health concerns, including strep throat. In this chapter, I will delve deeper into the fascinating world of acupuncture and acupressure, exploring their scientific basis, specific applications for strep throat symptoms, and their benefits for overall wellbeing.

Acupuncture and acupressure are both based on the concept of meridians, which are energy pathways that flow throughout the body. The underlying philosophy is that when these meridians are obstructed or imbalanced, it can lead to various health issues. Acupuncture involves the insertion of tiny needles into specific points along the meridians to restore the flow of energy, or qi, and stimulate the body's natural healing process. Acupressure, on the other hand, uses targeted pressure on these points to achieve similar effects. Both modalities aim to restore harmony and balance to the body.

Scientifically, acupuncture and acupressure have been shown to have profound effects on the nervous system, immune system, and hormonal balance. The insertion of acupuncture needles stimulates the release of endorphins, serotonin, and other neurotransmitters that help modulate pain signals and promote relaxation. This reduction in pain and stress can be particularly beneficial for strep throat, which is characterized by severe throat pain and inflammation.

Moreover, acupuncture has been found to enhance the immune response, helping the body fight off infections more effectively. Specific acupuncture points can boost the immune system, reduce inflammation, and increase blood circulation, promoting faster healing and alleviating strep throat symptoms such as sore throat, difficulty swallowing, and swollen lymph nodes. By addressing these symptoms at their root cause, acupuncture offers a holistic approach to strep throat management.

For those who prefer a non-invasive alternative, acupressure can provide similar benefits. By applying pressure to specific points, such as LI4 (Hegu) and LU11 (Shaoshang), individuals can experience relief from sore throat, reduce congestion, and support the body's natural healing processes. It is important to note that acupressure should be done with a gentle, steady pressure and should not cause pain or discomfort.

Beyond specifically addressing strep throat symptoms, acupuncture and acupressure offer a wide range of holistic benefits. These modalities can help reduce stress, improve sleep quality, enhance energy levels, and support the body's overall wellbeing. By restoring balance to the body's energy flow, individuals may experience improved mood, enhanced immune function, and a sense of overall vitality.

It is crucial to integrate acupuncture and acupressure with conventional medical treatment for strep throat. These modalities can complement traditional therapies, such as antibiotics, by speeding up the recovery process, reducing the severity of symptoms, and preventing recurrences. It is always recommended to consult with a qualified and licensed acupuncturist or practitioner to ensure the safest and most effective treatment.

Before considering acupuncture or acupressure for strep throat, there are some considerations and precautions to keep in mind. Individuals with certain medical conditions, such as bleeding disorders or pacemakers, should seek professional advice before undergoing acupuncture. Additionally, it is essential to choose a reputable practitioner who has the necessary training and experience. Potential side effects, such as minor bruising or soreness at the needle insertion sites, are rare, but it is important to discuss any concerns with the practitioner beforehand.

To further illustrate the effectiveness of acupuncture and acupressure for strep throat, I would like to share some personal testimonials and success stories. Many of my patients have found relief from their strep throat symptoms and experienced a significant improvement in their overall wellbeing after incorporating these modalities into their treatment plan. Their stories serve as a testament to the power of these ancient healing techniques.

In conclusion, acupuncture and acupressure offer a unique and holistic approach to addressing strep throat symptoms. By restoring balance and promoting the body's natural healing abilities, these modalities can provide relief from pain, reduce inflammation, and support overall wellbeing. Integrating acupuncture and acupressure with conventional medical treatment can enhance the effectiveness of both approaches and accelerate the recovery process. When considering acupuncture or acupressure, it is essential to seek professional advice and choose a qualified practitioner. With proper care and guidance, these ancient healing techniques can bring significant benefits to those suffering from strep throat.

Herbal Medicine and Supplements

Herbal medicine and supplements have long been used as natural remedies for various ailments, including strep throat. This alternative approach to healthcare focuses on harnessing the power of plants and natural ingredients to support the body's healing processes. In the context of strep throat, herbal medicine and supplements can play a significant role in boosting the immune system, reducing inflammation, and alleviating symptoms.

One of the key benefits of herbal medicine is its ability to strengthen the immune system. Certain herbs, such as echinacea, elderberry, and astragalus, are known for their immune-supporting properties. These herbs can help fortify the body's natural defenses, making it more resilient against bacteria and viruses that cause strep throat. By incorporating these immune-supporting herbs into your treatment plan, you can potentially reduce the severity and duration of your strep throat symptoms.

In addition to immune support, herbal medicine also offers specific benefits for strep throat management. For example, certain herbs have anti-inflammatory properties that can help reduce the swelling and pain associated with strep throat. Herbs like sage, thyme, and licorice root have been traditionally used to alleviate throat discomfort and soothe inflammation.

When it comes to herbal remedies for strep throat, there are several options available. These remedies can be prepared in various forms, including teas, gargles, and throat sprays. For example, you can make a sage tea by steeping dried sage leaves in hot water and then gargling with the liquid to help relieve throat pain and inflammation. Thyme can be prepared similarly, either in tea or gargle form, to help fight bacterial infections and reduce inflammation.

Supplements also play a role in supporting the immune system during strep throat recovery. Vitamins and minerals such as vitamin C and zinc are known for their immune-boosting properties. These can be taken as supplements to help strengthen the body's defenses. Probiotics, which promote a healthy gut microbiome, can also be beneficial in maintaining a strong immune system.

While herbal medicine and supplements can be advantageous, it is essential to consult with a healthcare professional before incorporating them into your treatment plan. They can guide you on the appropriate dosage, potential interactions with other medications, and any contraindications. It is important to remember that herbal medicine and supplements should complement conventional medical treatments rather than replace them.

To effectively incorporate herbal medicine and supplements into your strep throat recovery, it is helpful to follow a few tips. Firstly, ensure that you are using high-quality, reputable products. Look for supplements that are tested for purity and potency. Secondly, follow the recommended dosage instructions provided by the manufacturer or your healthcare professional. Consistency and regularity are key to experiencing the benefits of these natural remedies. Lastly, be mindful of any potential side effects or allergic reactions. If you experience any adverse effects, discontinue use and consult with your healthcare professional.

Research and evidence supporting the use of herbal medicine and supplements for strep throat recovery is constantly growing. Clinical trials, scientific studies, and anecdotal evidence collectively suggest that these natural remedies can provide significant benefits. However, it is important to note that individual results may vary, and the effectiveness of herbal medicine and supplements may depend on several factors, such as the severity of the infection and the individual's overall health.

In conclusion, herbal medicine and supplements offer a holistic approach to strep throat management by supporting the immune system, reducing inflammation, and alleviating symptoms. When used alongside conventional medical treatments, they can enhance the recovery process and promote overall well-being. However, it is crucial to seek guidance from a healthcare professional and be mindful of potential side effects or interactions. By incorporating herbal medicine and supplements into your strep throat recovery plan, you can empower your body's natural healing abilities and optimize your health and wellness.

Aromatherapy and Essential Oils

Introduction to aromatherapy and essential oils:

Aromatherapy is a branch of alternative medicine that utilizes the therapeutic properties of essential oils to promote physical and emotional well-being. Essential oils are highly concentrated plant extracts that capture the aromatic and healing essence of various plants. These oils are extracted through methods such as steam distillation or cold pressing, ensuring that they retain the beneficial properties of the plant.

In recent years, aromatherapy has gained significant popularity as a complementary therapy for various health conditions, including strep throat. The use of essential oils in aromatherapy can help alleviate symptoms such as sore throat, cough, and congestion, while also boosting mood and providing a sense of relaxation.

Understanding essential oils:

Essential oils are derived from different parts of various plants, including flowers, leaves, bark, and roots. They contain the natural compounds responsible for the plant's fragrance and medicinal properties. The concentration of these compounds in essential oils is significantly higher than in the plant itself, making them potent remedies for numerous ailments.

To ensure maximum effectiveness, it is crucial to use high-quality, pure essential oils. Inferior products may contain synthetic ingredients, which could be harmful or cause adverse reactions. When looking for essential oils, always check for labels indicating that they are 100% pure and therapeutic grade.

Benefits of aromatherapy for strep throat symptoms:

Aromatherapy can provide relief from the discomfort caused by strep throat symptoms. Several essential oils possess properties that can help alleviate inflammation, fight off microbial infections, and ease congestion.

Tea tree oil, for example, is well-known for its antimicrobial properties. It can help combat the bacterial infection causing strep throat, while also reducing inflammation and soothing a sore throat. Eucalyptus oil, with its expectorant properties, can assist in breaking up mucus and clearing congestion. Additionally, lavender oil has both anti-inflammatory and relaxing properties, which can aid in reducing discomfort and promoting restful sleep.

Aromatherapy techniques for strep throat relief:

There are various ways to incorporate aromatherapy into your strep throat recovery plan. Inhalation is a popular and effective method, as it allows the essential oils to reach the respiratory system directly. You can add a few drops of essential oil to a diffuser or vaporizer and inhale the scented steam. Alternatively, you can also add a few drops to a bowl of hot water and inhale the steam by placing a towel over your head.

Steam inhalation is particularly effective in soothing a sore throat and relieving congestion. Gargling with a diluted solution of essential oils mixed with warm water can also help alleviate throat discomfort. Remember to use essential oils in moderation and following appropriate dilution guidelines to avoid any adverse reactions.

Role of essential oils in boosting mood:

In addition to their physical benefits, certain essential oils can also enhance mood, promote relaxation, and reduce stress. Citrus oils such as lemon and orange are known for their uplifting and energizing properties, while floral oils like rose and ylang-ylang can help create a soothing and calming atmosphere.

During the strep throat recovery process, incorporating these mood-boosting essential oils into your aromatherapy practices can have a positive impact on your overall well-being. By creating an environment that supports a positive mindset, you can enhance your body's natural healing abilities.

Aromatherapy safety considerations:

While aromatherapy and essential oils are generally safe when used correctly, it is essential to exercise caution and seek guidance from a qualified aromatherapist or healthcare professional. This is especially important if you have underlying health conditions or are taking medications, as certain essential oils may interact with medications or exacerbate certain health conditions.

Before using any essential oils, ensure that you are aware of proper dilution techniques and usage guidelines. Some essential oils may cause skin sensitivities or allergic reactions, so a patch test on a small area of the skin is recommended before widespread use.

Conclusion to the subchapter:

In conclusion, aromatherapy and essential oils offer a natural and holistic approach to relieving strep throat symptoms and promoting well-being. By utilizing the therapeutic properties of essential oils, such as their antimicrobial, anti-inflammatory, and mood-enhancing properties, you can enhance the strep throat recovery process. However, it is important to remember that further research and evidence are necessary to fully understand the effectiveness of aromatherapy for strep throat. Aromatherapy should complement conventional medical treatments and be used with caution, ensuring the safety and well-being of the individual.

Mind-Body Therapies

The concept of mind-body therapies is an invaluable approach to managing strep throat that emphasizes the vital connection between the mind and body. When we focus on relaxation and harness the power of our mind, we can significantly impact our physical well-being and effectively manage symptoms of strep throat. Mind-body therapies encompass a range of practices and techniques that promote holistic healthcare and wellness. These therapies aim to not only alleviate physical symptoms but also enhance emotional well-being, increase resilience, and support the body's natural healing processes.

One example of a mind-body therapy that can be particularly beneficial for strep throat management is yoga. Yoga is a practice that combines various physical poses, breathing exercises, and meditation techniques to promote relaxation, balance, and overall well-being. When it comes to strep throat, specific yoga poses and breathing exercises can help alleviate symptoms and enhance recovery. Poses such as the Child's Pose, which involves kneeling and resting the forehead on the floor while stretching the arms forward, can help soothe and relieve discomfort in the throat. Additionally, deep breathing exercises, such as Alternate Nostril Breathing, can support respiratory health and improve oxygenation in the body. By regularly incorporating yoga into a strep throat treatment plan, patients can experience not only physical relief but also a sense of calm and centeredness that aids in the healing process.

Another powerful mind-body therapy that can complement strep throat management is guided imagery. Guided imagery involves consciously creating mental images to promote relaxation and alleviate symptoms. By visualizing calming and healing scenarios, individuals can create a sense of peace and facilitate the body's natural healing response. For strep throat patients, guided imagery exercises can be specifically adapted to target throat discomfort and promote healing.

For example, an imagery exercise may involve visualizing a soothing, golden light enveloping the throat and gently restoring it to health and vibrancy. By exploring guided imagery as a complementary therapy, strep throat patients can tap into the potential benefits of visualization and harness the mind's power to support their physical well-being.

Integrating mind-body therapies into a comprehensive treatment plan for strep throat is essential for optimal results. It is crucial to engage in open and honest conversations with healthcare professionals and receive guidance on how to effectively incorporate mind-body techniques. By working collaboratively with a healthcare team, patients can ensure that mind-body therapies are integrated safely and effectively into their overall care. Combining mind-body therapies with conventional medical treatments can provide a holistic and comprehensive approach to strep throat management, addressing both the physical and emotional aspects of the condition.

Scientific research and evidence support the efficacy of mind-body therapies in strep throat management. Numerous studies have demonstrated the positive impact of practices like yoga and guided imagery on reducing inflammation, alleviating symptoms, and supporting overall well-being. By exploring the research evidence, patients can feel confident in the effectiveness and evidence-based nature of mind-body therapies. This knowledge empowers individuals to take an active role in their own health and well-being and make informed decisions about their treatment options.

Stress reduction is a key aspect of managing strep throat, as stress can exacerbate symptoms and hinder the healing process. Mind-body therapies play a crucial role in reducing stress levels and promoting emotional well-being. By engaging in practices like yoga, guided imagery, and other relaxation techniques, patients can effectively manage stress and create a positive environment for healing. When stress levels are reduced, the body's immune system is strengthened, allowing for a faster recovery and a smoother healing process.

Incorporating mind-body therapies into one's daily routine requires consistency and commitment. Practical tips and suggestions can help individuals integrate these therapies seamlessly into their lives. For example, setting aside dedicated time each day for yoga or guided imagery exercises can create a regular practice that becomes a natural part of one's routine. It is important to prioritize self-care and make mind-body therapies a priority, just like any other aspect of wellness. By dedicating time and energy to these practices, strep throat patients can reap the significant benefits for their overall well-being.

In addition to yoga and guided imagery, there are various other mind-body therapies that strep throat patients can explore. Practices such as meditation, relaxation techniques, and mindfulness can further support relaxation, stress reduction, and emotional well-being. Each individual may resonate with different therapies, and it is important to explore and find what works best for one's unique needs and preferences. Mind-body therapies offer a diverse range of options that empower individuals to take an active role in their healing journey.

Real-life case studies and personal stories can serve as powerful inspiration for strep throat patients considering mind-body therapies. Hearing about the experiences and outcomes of others who have successfully incorporated these therapies into their treatment plans can provide valuable insights and motivation. These personal stories validate the effectiveness and potential of mind-body therapies and offer hope and encouragement to those embarking on their own healing journey. By sharing and learning from these experiences, patients can build confidence and trust in the benefits of mind-body therapies.

As the field of mind-body therapies continues to evolve, it is important to stay curious and open to new advancements and possibilities. The future of mind-body therapies for strep throat management may include technology-assisted therapies or innovative approaches that further enhance relaxation, well-being, and healing. By embracing a mindset of curiosity and possibility, strep throat patients can actively engage in their treatment and remain open to new avenues of support and healing.

In conclusion, mind-body therapies offer a comprehensive and holistic approach to managing strep throat. By integrating practices such as yoga, guided imagery, and other relaxation techniques into a treatment plan, patients can tap into the incredible power of their mind to support their physical well-being. These therapies not only alleviate symptoms but also promote emotional well-being, stress reduction, and overall wellness. By exploring mind-body therapies, patients become active participants in their healing journey, enhancing their resilience and well-being.

Chapter 5: Psychological Support for Strep Throat Patients

Emotional Impact of Strep Throat

In the midst of battling the physical symptoms of strep throat, it is essential to recognize and address the emotional impact that this condition can have on patients. As a medical doctor and health and wellness coach, I have witnessed firsthand the profound effect that strep throat can have on individuals' emotional well-being. Understanding and addressing these emotional challenges is crucial for patients' overall well-being and healing process.

Frustration often accompanies the experience of strep throat. The physical symptoms, such as the persistent throat pain and difficulty swallowing, can be incredibly frustrating. Simple tasks like eating, drinking, and even speaking become arduous challenges, leading to an overwhelming sense of helplessness. As a result, patients may feel a deep sense of frustration and irritability, as their bodies seem to betray them. The inability to engage in usual activities and routines due to illness further intensifies this frustration, leading to feelings of being trapped and limited.

Anxiety also tends to weave its way into the emotional landscape of strep throat patients. The fear and worry associated with the illness can be overwhelming. Concerns about the recovery process, potential complications, and the impact on daily life can consume one's thoughts. The uncertainty surrounding the healing process and the duration of the illness can also trigger heightened anxiety. These anxious thoughts and fears can exacerbate physical symptoms and make the recovery process more challenging.

Feelings of isolation often plague those affected by strep throat. As a contagious illness, patients must isolate themselves from others to prevent spreading the infection. This necessary precaution, while crucial, can create a deep sense of loneliness and disconnection. The loss of social support and the absence of physical contact can take a toll on mental well-being, leading to feelings of sadness and even depression. The inability to participate in social activities, including work, school, and social gatherings, can further intensify these feelings of isolation.

Recognizing and addressing the emotional challenges that accompany strep throat is essential for patients' overall well-being. Here are some strategies and techniques to help manage the frustration, anxiety, and feelings of isolation that often arise:

1. Patience and Self-compassion: Practicing patience and being self-compassionate during the recovery process can help alleviate frustration. Understand that healing takes time, and it is okay to prioritize rest and self-care.

2. Support from Loved Ones: Seek support from friends, family, and loved ones. Communicate your feelings and let them know how they can help during this difficult time. Sometimes, a listening ear and empathetic presence can work wonders in lifting one's spirits.

3. Stress-reducing Activities: Engage in stress-reducing activities that bring joy and help to distract from the discomforts of strep throat. This can include activities such as reading, listening to music, practicing relaxation techniques like guided imagery, or pursuing hobbies.

4. Deep Breathing and Mindfulness: Incorporate deep breathing exercises and mindfulness techniques into your daily routine. These practices can help calm the mind, reduce anxiety, and promote emotional well-being.

5. Professional Support: If feelings of anxiety or depression become overwhelming, do not hesitate to seek professional support. A therapist or counselor can provide guidance and support in navigating the emotional challenges that arise during strep throat.

6. Staying Connected: While physical isolation is necessary, staying connected with others through technology can alleviate feelings of loneliness. Utilize platforms like video calls and social media to stay in touch with loved ones and maintain a sense of social connection.

7. Online Communities: Seek support from online communities that focus on strep throat or other individuals going through similar health challenges. Sharing experiences, seeking advice, and connecting with others who understand can help combat feelings of isolation and provide a sense of camaraderie.

Addressing the emotional impact of strep throat is integral to the comprehensive management of this condition. By acknowledging and supporting patients' emotional well-being, not only do we alleviate their suffering, but we also foster an environment conducive to physical healing and recovery. Integrating emotional wellness into the management of strep throat empowers patients to navigate the ups and downs of their journey towards wellness more effectively.

As we move forward in this book, we will delve deeper into self-care techniques specifically tailored for strep throat patients. We will explore how lifestyle modifications, dietary changes, and holistic approaches can aid in the healing process. By addressing not only the physical symptoms but also the emotional and mental aspects of strep throat, we can help patients achieve a comprehensive state of well-being. Join me in the next chapter as we dive into the empowering world of self-care strategies for strep throat.

Cognitive Behavioral Therapy (CBT)

In my years of practice as a medical doctor and health and wellness coach, I have witnessed firsthand the profound impact that Cognitive Behavioral Therapy (CBT) can have on the emotional well-being of strep throat patients. CBT is a powerful therapeutic approach that aims to manage negative thoughts and emotions by challenging and modifying cognitive distortions, ultimately leading to positive changes in behavior and overall well-being.

To truly understand the benefits of CBT, it is important to explore the relationship between thoughts, emotions, and strep throat. When we experience negative thoughts and emotions, such as frustration, anxiety, and isolation, it can exacerbate the physical symptoms of strep throat and impede the healing process. By addressing these psychological factors, we can provide patients with a holistic approach to their recovery journey.

The first step in CBT is identifying negative thoughts and emotions. Often, these thoughts can be distorted and exaggerated, leading to heightened negative emotions. By recognizing these patterns, patients can actively challenge and reframe their thoughts into more realistic and positive ones. This process can be achieved through thought records, which allow patients to examine their thoughts and the evidence supporting them.

Behavioral activation is another crucial component of CBT. Engaging in positive and enjoyable activities can improve mood and overall well-being, countering the negative effects of strep throat. Encouraging patients to pursue activities they love and find purpose in is essential, as it provides a sense of fulfillment and distraction from the discomforts of their condition.

In addition to behavioral activation, relaxation and stress management techniques play a vital role in improving negative thoughts and emotions associated with strep throat. Deep breathing exercises, progressive muscle relaxation, and mindfulness meditation can effectively calm the mind, reduce anxiety, and promote emotional well-being. These techniques enable patients to cultivate a sense of inner peace amid the challenges they face.

Problem-solving skills are crucial in managing the hurdles that are often encountered during strep throat recovery. By developing effective problem-solving techniques, patients can identify the problems they face, generate practical solutions, and implement them effectively. This empowers patients to regain a sense of control and lessen feelings of frustration and helplessness.

Cognitive restructuring is a fundamental technique in CBT that involves challenging and replacing negative thoughts with more positive and rational ones. By examining the evidence supporting negative thoughts and questioning their accuracy, patients can reframe their thoughts into a healthier and more empowering mindset. This process ultimately leads to a more positive outlook on their recovery journey.

Maintaining the positive changes achieved through CBT is essential for long-term well-being. Integrating these techniques into daily life ensures that patients continue managing their thoughts and emotions associated with strep throat even after their recovery. It is important to make self-care a priority, making time for activities that bring joy, practicing stress management techniques regularly, and seeking support from loved ones.

Of course, there may be times when professional help is needed. Therapists or counselors trained in CBT can provide additional guidance and support in navigating the challenges of strep throat recovery. Seeking their assistance can enhance patients' understanding and application of CBT principles and techniques, ultimately leading to a more successful and comprehensive recovery.

As we progress further in this book, we will explore self-care techniques specifically tailored for strep throat patients. By addressing not only the physical symptoms but also the emotional and mental aspects of strep throat, we can empower patients to navigate their journey towards wellness more effectively. Join me in the next chapter as we dive into the empowering world of self-care strategies for strep throat.

Building a Support System

Introduction to the importance of a strong support system

A strong support system is crucial for anyone facing the challenges of strep throat. This network of support can provide comfort, motivation, and guidance throughout the recovery process. Whether it is emotional support from loved ones or professional advice from healthcare providers, building a support system plays a vital role in ensuring the patient's overall well-being. In this chapter, we will delve deeper into the different aspects of building a support system and explore how it can positively impact the journey to recovery.

Importance of emotional support from friends and family

During times of illness, the emotional support of friends and family members can be an invaluable source of strength. Simply knowing that there are loved ones who care deeply for you can provide comfort and solace during the trying days of strep throat recovery. They can be a listening ear, offering empathy and understanding, and lighten the emotional burden that often comes with being unwell.

Friends and family also serve as a source of encouragement. Their words of affirmation and positivity can motivate the patient to stay resilient and focused on their recovery goals. Whether it is a small victory like completing a day of medication or a setback that requires a shift in treatment plans, the unwavering support of loved ones can provide the much-needed boost to keep the patient going.

Seek support from healthcare professionals

In addition to the support of friends and family, it is essential to seek guidance from healthcare professionals who specialize in treating strep throat. These professionals possess deep knowledge and experience in managing the condition and can offer valuable medical advice and guidance throughout the recovery process.

Finding the right healthcare professional can be a daunting task, but it is crucial to identify someone who understands the specific challenges that strep throat patients face. Look for professionals who are compassionate, knowledgeable, and have a holistic approach to healthcare. By seeking their support, patients can rest assured that they are receiving the optimal treatment and care for their condition.

Effective communication with your support system

Building a strong support system requires open and honest communication. It is important to express your needs, concerns, and fears to your friends, family, and healthcare professionals. By sharing your thoughts and emotions, you enable them to provide the most appropriate support and guidance.

Effective communication techniques can facilitate this process. Active listening, for example, allows you to truly hear what others are saying and validate their experiences. On the other hand, assertive communication empowers you to express your needs and concerns in a respectful manner, while also setting boundaries when necessary. By developing these skills, you pave the way for genuine and meaningful connections within your support system.

Understanding the different roles of your support system members

Friends, family, and healthcare professionals each play a unique role in the support system. Friends and family provide emotional support, but they can also help with practical matters, such as assisting with daily activities or coordinating medical appointments. Healthcare professionals, on the other hand, offer medical expertise and treatment options that are tailored to your specific needs.

Recognizing these different roles is important in order to fully benefit from the support system. By understanding what each member brings to the table, you can effectively utilize their strengths and expertise to enhance your overall well-being.

Building a support network beyond friends and family

While friends and family are invaluable sources of support, it can also be beneficial to expand your network beyond immediate loved ones. Joining support groups or online communities for strep throat patients can provide a sense of belonging and connection with others who are going through similar experiences. These communities offer a platform to share experiences, exchange coping strategies, and offer encouragement to one another. By connecting with like-minded individuals, you can broaden your support system and gain additional perspectives on managing strep throat.

Addressing potential challenges in building a support system

Building a support system is not without its challenges. Busy schedules, geographical distances, or family dynamics can pose obstacles to establishing and maintaining a robust support network. However, it is important to recognize these challenges and develop strategies to overcome them.

Setting boundaries is crucial in managing these challenges. Communicate your needs and limitations to your support system members, ensuring that you have the necessary space and time for your own self-care. If needed, do not hesitate to seek professional help to navigate these challenges. Therapists or counselors can provide guidance and support in managing interpersonal dynamics or improving communication within your support system.

Seek professional counseling or therapy if necessary

Sometimes, strep throat recovery can bring about emotional and psychological challenges that require professional assistance. If you find yourself feeling overwhelmed or struggling to cope, reaching out for professional counseling or therapy can be immensely helpful. These professionals are trained to address the emotional and mental aspects of strep throat recovery and can provide guidance on developing coping strategies and enhancing resilience.

The impact of a strong support system on overall well-being

Having a strong support system can positively impact a patient's mental, emotional, and physical well-being. Emotional support from friends and family can alleviate stress, anxiety, and feelings of isolation. Professional guidance ensures that patients receive the best medical care and advice. By taking advantage of the resources available within their support system, patients can experience improved overall well-being and a more effective recovery from strep throat.

In conclusion, building a strong support system is vital for anyone facing the challenges of strep throat. Emotional support from loved ones, guidance from healthcare professionals, and active communication within the support system all contribute to the patient's well-being. By actively seeking and nurturing a support network, patients can empower themselves to navigate their strep throat recovery with resilience and positivity.

Maintaining a Positive Mindset

Introduction to Maintaining a Positive Mindset

Throughout your strep throat journey, maintaining a positive mindset holds immense power. It acts as a guiding force, motivating you to persevere and promoting overall well-being during the recovery process. When faced with the challenges of strep throat, a positive mindset becomes your strongest ally, empowering you to navigate the ups and downs with resilience and grace. By embracing positivity, you can unlock your inner strength and approach your recovery with a renewed sense of hope and determination.

The Power of Positive Thinking

Positive thinking goes beyond mere optimism. It is a mindset that focuses on recognizing and embracing the potential for growth and healing even amidst adversity. By cultivating positive thoughts, you can harness the healing power of your mind and impact both your physical and mental health. Scientific research has shown that positive thinking can lower stress levels, enhance immune function, promote faster recovery, and increase overall well-being. By adopting a positive mindset, you are not only supporting your body's healing processes but also nurturing your emotional well-being.

Cultivating Resilience

Resilience is the ability to bounce back from setbacks, to adapt, and to thrive in the face of challenges. Strengthening your resilience is crucial throughout the strep throat journey, as it helps you overcome hurdles and maintain a positive mindset. Cultivating resilience requires practicing self-care, developing coping strategies, and nurturing an unwavering belief in your ability to overcome obstacles. By embracing resilience, you can transform setbacks into opportunities for growth, emergence, and ultimate triumph over strep throat.

Daily Affirmations

Affirmations are powerful tools for maintaining a positive mindset. By repeating positive statements, you can rewire your subconscious mind, reinforce your self-belief, and boost your confidence. During your strep throat journey, affirmations can be tailored to uplift and support you, acting as constant reminders of your inner strength and resilience. Some examples of affirmations include, "I am healing with each passing day," "I am strong and capable of overcoming any challenge," and "I am deserving of love, care, and well-being." Implementing daily affirmations can have transformative effects on your mindset and foster a sense of empowerment.

Mindfulness and Meditation

Mindfulness and meditation are practices that cultivate a deep sense of presence and awareness. By giving your full attention to the present moment, you can reduce stress, anxiety, and negative thinking patterns, while nurturing a positive mindset. Mindfulness involves letting go of judgments and embracing acceptance, allowing you to navigate the strep throat journey with compassion for yourself and others. Meditation, on the other hand, provides an opportunity to quiet the mind, find inner peace, and connect with a deeper sense of purpose. Incorporating mindfulness and meditation into your daily routine can promote relaxation, clarity, and a positive outlook.

Gratitude Practice

Practicing gratitude involves intentionally focusing on the blessings and positive aspects of your life, even amidst the challenges of strep throat. By shifting your attention to what you are grateful for, you cultivate a positive mindset and enhance your overall well-being. Gratitude practice can take many forms, such as keeping a gratitude journal, verbally expressing gratitude to loved ones, or simply taking a moment each day to reflect on the things that bring you joy and appreciation. By acknowledging and appreciating the small joys and blessings in your life, you amplify positivity and strengthen your inner resilience.

Social Support and Connection

Building a strong support system is vital for maintaining a positive mindset throughout your strep throat journey. Seeking support from friends, family, or support groups can provide a sense of belonging, empathy, and encouragement. Sharing your experiences and emotions with others who understand can lift your spirits and remind you that you are not alone. Connecting with individuals who have gone through similar challenges can offer valuable insights, coping strategies, and inspiration. By nurturing social support and connection, you build a network of care that can uplift and inspire you while fostering a positive mindset.

Managing Stress and Anxiety

Strep throat can bring about stress and anxiety, affecting both your physical and mental well-being. It is important to develop effective techniques for managing these challenging emotions during your recovery journey. Engaging in relaxation techniques such as deep breathing exercises, progressive muscle relaxation, or guided imagery can help calm your mind and release tension from your body. Additionally, incorporating stress management strategies such as time management, prioritizing self-care, and setting healthy boundaries can alleviate stress and support a positive mindset. By actively managing stress and anxiety, you empower yourself to navigate the strep throat journey with resilience and clarity.

Positive Visualization

Positive visualization is a practice that involves picturing your desired outcome and envisioning your journey to healing and recovery. By visualizing yourself healthy, vibrant, and free from strep throat, you can positively impact your mindset and support your body's innate healing abilities. Visualize the progression of your recovery, from the first signs of improvement to complete wellness. Engaging in positive visualization regularly can inspire hope, cultivate optimism, and strengthen your commitment to maintaining a positive mindset throughout the strep throat journey.

Self-Care Practices for Mental Well-being

Prioritizing self-care is crucial for nurturing a positive mindset during your strep throat recovery. Engaging in activities that bring you joy, relaxation, and fulfillment can enhance your mental well-being and promote a positive outlook. Take time to indulge in hobbies, connect with nature, practice self-compassion, or engage in creative outlets. Ensuring that your emotional and mental needs are met through self-care practices fosters resilience, self-empowerment, and a profound sense of well-being.

Overcoming Setbacks and Challenges

The strep throat journey may not always be smooth sailing. Setbacks and challenges can arise, testing your resilience and commitment to maintaining a positive mindset. However, setbacks can also be valuable opportunities for growth and learning. Embrace setbacks as temporary obstacles rather than permanent failures, and adopt a mindset of perseverance and resilience. By reframing challenges as stepping stones, you can overcome obstacles with courage, determination, and unwavering optimism.

Harnessing the Power of Positive Affirmations

Positive affirmations are not just mere words; they hold immense power when created with intention and belief. Take time to create personalized affirmations that resonate with your strep throat journey, reflecting your specific goals, strengths, and aspirations. Repeat these affirmations daily, embedding them deeply within your subconscious mind. When you truly believe in the power of your affirmations, you unleash your inner potential and propel yourself towards a more positive path of healing and well-being.

Celebrating Progress and Achievements

Recognizing and celebrating your progress, no matter how small, is essential for maintaining a positive mindset. Each step forward, each sign of improvement deserves acknowledgement and celebration. Take time to reflect on your accomplishments, however small they may seem. Whether it's your first bite of solid food or a day without a fever, celebrate each milestone as a victory on your strep throat journey. By celebrating progress and achievements, you reinforce your positive mindset, boost your motivation, and cultivate a sense of satisfaction and gratitude.

Finding Meaning and Purpose

Finding meaning and purpose in your strep throat journey can significantly impact your mindset and overall well-being. Reflect on how this experience has shaped you, what you have learned, and what values you prioritize. Consider how you can align your life with these values, even during the recovery process. Engaging in activities that bring you joy, fulfillment, and a sense of purpose can nurture your positive mindset and help you navigate the strep throat journey with a deeper sense of meaning.

Embracing Positivity in Daily Life

A positive mindset is not limited to the strep throat journey; it is a way of life. Extend your positive mindset beyond recovery and integrate it into your daily life. Embrace positivity in all aspects of life, including work, relationships, and self-care. Practice gratitude, resilience, and self-compassion in your everyday interactions. By consciously choosing to approach life with positivity and a resilient mindset, you foster long-term well-being and a profound sense of self-empowerment.

Conclusion

Maintaining a positive mindset throughout your strep throat journey is a transformative and empowering endeavor. By harnessing the power of positive thinking, cultivating resilience, engaging in daily affirmations, practicing mindfulness and gratitude, seeking social support, managing stress and anxiety, harnessing the power of visualization, prioritizing self-care, and celebrating progress, you can navigate your strep throat journey with unwavering optimism. Embrace the possibilities that a positive mindset brings, nurture your inner resilience, and empower yourself to overcome the challenges of strep throat with grace and determination. Remember, your mindset has the potential to shape your reality, and with a positive mindset, you can rewrite your strep throat story filled with hope, healing, and well-being.

Chapter 6: Long-Term Management and Prevention

Recurrence Prevention

Recurrence prevention is a crucial aspect of managing strep throat in order to minimize the frequency of its occurrence. By implementing effective strategies, we can significantly reduce the chances of experiencing multiple episodes of strep throat and its associated discomfort. Maintaining good hygiene practices and bolstering the immune system play vital roles in preventing the recurrence of this condition.

Good hygiene practices are essential to combating the spread and recurrence of strep throat. Regular handwashing is paramount, ensuring that we scrub our hands for at least twenty seconds with soap and water, especially before and after meals, after using the restroom, and after coming into contact with any potentially contaminated surfaces. It is equally important to practice proper coughing and sneezing etiquette, such as covering our mouths and noses with a tissue or our elbow to prevent the spread of infectious droplets. Regularly disinfecting frequently touched surfaces, such as doorknobs, light switches, and shared electronic devices, can further minimize the risk of strep throat recurrence.

Boosting the immune system is another key component in preventing strep throat recurrence. A healthy immune system is our body's natural defense against infections, including strep throat. It is crucial to prioritize a nutrient-rich diet, comprising a variety of fruits, vegetables, whole grains, lean proteins, and healthy fats. These foods provide the vitamins, minerals, and antioxidants necessary for optimal immune function. Regular exercise not only helps to strengthen the immune system but also improves circulation, which aids in the removal of toxins and supports overall health. Adequate sleep is equally vital, as it allows our bodies to repair and replenish immune cells. Furthermore, incorporating immune-boosting supplements or herbs, such as vitamin C, zinc, garlic, echinacea, or elderberry, into our routine can provide an added immune system reinforcement.

Nutrition plays a significant role in preventing strep throat recurrence. Including specific foods known for their immune-boosting properties can notably support our body's defense against infections. Citrus fruits and berries are rich in vitamin C, a potent antioxidant that enhances immune function. Leafy green vegetables, such as spinach and kale, are abundant in vitamins A, C, and E, as well as other essential nutrients that support immune health. Probiotic foods, such as yogurt and fermented vegetables, promote a healthy gut microbiome, which is closely linked to immune function. Additionally, incorporating foods rich in zinc, such as legumes, nuts, and seeds, can further strengthen the immune system and protect against strep throat recurrence.

In addition to practicing good hygiene, boosting the immune system, and maintaining a nutrient-rich diet, there are other measures we can take to prevent the recurrence of strep throat. Minimizing close contact with individuals currently experiencing a strep throat infection, especially in crowded settings, can reduce our exposure to the bacteria. Moreover, maintaining a clean and healthy living environment, regularly disinfecting surfaces, and frequently washing bedding and towels can further prevent the spread and recurrence of strep throat. It is crucial to be proactive in seeking regular medical check-ups to monitor for any signs of strep throat recurrence and promptly address any potential underlying health conditions that may contribute to its occurrence.

The role of stress management cannot be overlooked when considering the prevention of strep throat recurrence. Chronic stress can weaken the immune system, making it more susceptible to infections. Incorporating stress management techniques, such as meditation, mindfulness, or therapy, into our daily routine can significantly reduce stress levels and strengthen our immune system.

By effectively managing stress, we empower ourselves to better protect against the recurrence of strep throat.

Education and empowerment are vital aspects of preventing strep throat recurrence. By educating ourselves about the causes, symptoms, and prevention strategies of strep throat, we gain a better understanding of how to avoid its recurrence. Taking an active role in our own health by implementing recommended strategies and making informed decisions about our lifestyle and habits allows us to proactively prevent strep throat from reoccurring. We must develop a sense of agency over our health and take responsibility for our well-being.

Seeking support from healthcare professionals, support groups, or online communities can greatly assist us in preventing recurrence. Engaging with others who have experienced or are going through similar situations can provide valuable insight, advice, and encouragement. Support networks and available resources can empower us with the tools needed to prevent strep throat from reoccurring while offering guidance and support along the way.

In conclusion, recurrence prevention is a crucial aspect of managing strep throat. By implementing effective hygiene practices, boosting the immune system, maintaining a nutrient-rich diet, and taking additional preventive measures, such as avoiding close contact with infected individuals and managing stress, we can significantly reduce the likelihood of strep throat recurrence. Education, empowerment, and seeking support from healthcare professionals and others experiencing similar situations are also key components in our journey to prevent the reoccurrence of strep throat. By taking proactive measures and making informed decisions about our health, we set ourselves on a path towards a strep throat-free future.

Follow-up Care and Monitoring

Introduction to Follow-up Care and Monitoring:

Follow-up care and monitoring are essential components of strep throat management. It involves regular check-ups and assessments to ensure optimal recovery and to monitor the effectiveness of treatment. By consistently monitoring the patient's condition, healthcare professionals can make necessary adjustments to the treatment plan and address any concerns or complications that may arise. In this section, we will delve deeper into the importance of follow-up care and monitoring for strep throat patients.

The Role of Healthcare Professionals in Follow-up Care:

Healthcare professionals play a crucial role in providing follow-up care and monitoring for strep throat patients. With their expertise and knowledge, they can accurately assess symptoms, evaluate treatment outcomes, and make informed decisions regarding further management. By collaborating with patients, healthcare professionals can create a comprehensive and tailored approach to treatment and recovery. Through regular follow-up appointments, they can closely monitor the patient's progress and adjust the treatment plan based on their evolving needs.

Evaluating the Effectiveness of Treatment:

Follow-up care and monitoring allow healthcare professionals to evaluate the effectiveness of strep throat treatment. By closely monitoring symptoms, they can determine if the prescribed treatment is successfully addressing the infection. This evaluation is crucial in ensuring that the patient is responding well to the treatment and recovering optimally. If the treatment is not yielding the desired outcomes, healthcare professionals can explore alternative options and adjust the treatment plan accordingly.

Tracking Compliance with Treatment Plan:

One of the primary reasons for follow-up care and monitoring is to track patient compliance with the prescribed treatment plan. Adherence to the treatment plan is crucial for effective management and recovery from strep throat. Healthcare professionals closely monitor and encourage patient compliance during follow-up appointments. They may provide strategies, reminders, and educational resources to help patients stay on track with their treatment plan. This close monitoring ensures that the patient is receiving the necessary care and support for their recovery.

Identifying Potential Complications or Recurrence:

Regular follow-up care and monitoring help healthcare professionals identify potential complications or recurrences of strep throat. By closely observing the patient's symptoms and overall health during follow-up appointments, healthcare professionals can detect any signs of complications or recurrence. Early detection is vital for prompt intervention and prevention of further complications. Through regular monitoring, healthcare professionals can provide appropriate treatment and guidance to minimize the risk of complications or recurrence.

Addressing Patient Concerns and Questions:

Follow-up care and monitoring provide an opportunity for strep throat patients to address their concerns and ask questions. Healthcare professionals understand the importance of open communication and actively encourage patients to share any worries or queries they may have. By addressing these concerns and providing reassurance, education, and support, healthcare professionals can foster a sense of trust and empower patients to actively participate in their own recovery.

Preventive Measures and Future Planning:

Follow-up care and monitoring also play a critical role in preventive measures for strep throat. Healthcare professionals may recommend lifestyle modifications and preventative strategies to minimize the risk of recurrence. These measures may include practicing good hygiene, adapting a nutrient-rich diet, and implementing stress management techniques. Regular check-ups and monitoring appointments are scheduled to ensure long-term strep throat management and prevention.

The Role of Self-Monitoring and Self-Care:

Patients also have a crucial role to play in follow-up care and monitoring. Self-monitoring and self-care practices enable patients to track their symptoms, adherence to the treatment plan, and general well-being at home. By actively participating in their recovery, patients can take control of their health and contribute to the effectiveness of treatment. Healthcare professionals provide guidance, resources, and support to empower patients in their self-monitoring and self-care practices.

Collaborative Approach in Follow-up Care and Monitoring:

Follow-up care and monitoring are most successful with a collaborative approach between healthcare professionals and strep throat patients. By actively involving patients in their care, healthcare professionals benefit from their insights and feedback regarding their symptoms, treatment responses, and overall well-being. This collaborative approach enhances the patient's sense of agency and responsibility for their health, leading to more effective management and recovery from strep throat.

Importance of Regular Follow-up Care and Monitoring:

In conclusion, regular follow-up care and monitoring are crucial for strep throat management. It ensures optimal recovery, early detection of complications, and prevention of recurrence. By prioritizing follow-up appointments and actively engaging in self-monitoring and self-care practices, patients maximize their chances of a successful recovery. Through open communication and collaboration, healthcare professionals and patients work together to develop a comprehensive and personalized approach to strep throat management.

Healthy Lifestyle Habits

Introduction to Healthy Lifestyle Habits:

As we delve into the middle portion of this book, it is important to emphasize the vital role that healthy lifestyle habits play in managing strep throat. These habits not only support overall well-being, but they also reduce the risk of developing strep throat or experiencing recurrent episodes. In this subchapter, I will guide you through various aspects of a healthy lifestyle and how they can contribute to strep throat prevention and management. By incorporating these habits into your daily routine, you can bolster your body's defenses against strep throat and promote optimal health.

Eating a Balanced Diet:

A balanced diet is essential for maintaining a robust immune system, which is crucial in the management of strep throat. By nourishing our bodies with nutrient-rich foods, we provide them with the building blocks necessary for optimal immune function. Vitamins and minerals, such as vitamin C and zinc, play a particularly important role in bolstering the immune system. By regularly consuming a variety of fruits, vegetables, lean proteins, whole grains, and healthy fats, we can support overall health and reduce the risk of strep throat. Some examples of specific foods that can provide these immune-boosting nutrients include citrus fruits, nuts, seeds, dark leafy greens, and yogurt.

Regular Exercise:

Regular exercise offers numerous benefits for strep throat management. Not only does it enhance overall well-being, but it also strengthens the immune system. Engaging in moderate-intensity activities, such as brisk walking, cycling, or swimming, can improve immune function by increasing the circulation of immune cells throughout the body. Additionally, exercise promotes the release of endorphins, which can help to alleviate stress and enhance mood. By incorporating different types of exercises into your daily routine, such as cardiovascular workouts, strength training, and flexibility exercises, you can optimize your immune system and support your strep throat management efforts.

Adequate Sleep:

A good night's sleep is crucial for strep throat management. During sleep, our bodies repair and replenish, including our immune system. Sufficient sleep supports immune function by reducing inflammation in the body and supporting the production and activity of immune cells. It is recommended to aim for seven to nine hours of quality sleep each night. To improve sleep quality and establish a regular sleep routine, it is helpful to create a relaxing sleep environment, establish a bedtime routine, adopt relaxation techniques before bed, and limit exposure to electronic devices before sleep.

Hydration:

Staying hydrated is often overlooked but plays a significant role in strep throat management. Drinking an adequate amount of water throughout the day helps to maintain a healthy throat and prevent infections. Water supports the production of saliva, which contains enzymes that can neutralize harmful bacteria and viruses. It also helps to keep mucous membranes hydrated, enabling them to act as a protective barrier against pathogens. To increase daily water intake, practical tips include carrying a water bottle with you, setting reminders to drink water, and consuming hydrating foods such as fruits and vegetables.

Stress Management:

Chronic stress can have a detrimental impact on immune function, increasing the risk of developing strep throat. Therefore, it is crucial to incorporate stress management techniques into your daily routine. Mindfulness techniques, such as deep breathing exercises and meditation, can help alleviate stress and promote relaxation. Engaging in regular physical activity, practicing self-care activities, and seeking support from loved ones can also contribute to effective stress management. By finding balance and prioritizing self-care, you can reduce stress levels and enhance your overall strep throat management efforts.

Avoidance of Smoking and Alcohol:

Smoking and excessive alcohol consumption have well-documented negative effects on overall health and immune function. They can weaken the immune system, making individuals more susceptible to infections such as strep throat. Quitting smoking and reducing alcohol intake are valuable steps in strep throat management and improving overall well-being. Seek support from healthcare professionals, consider joining support groups, and explore alternative coping strategies to overcome these habits and prioritize your health.

Good Hygiene Practices:

Practicing good hygiene is essential in preventing the spread of strep throat. By following simple yet effective hygiene recommendations, we can minimize the risk of infection and maintain overall health. Regular and thorough handwashing with soap and water is crucial, especially before meals and after using the restroom. Additionally, covering the mouth and nose when coughing or sneezing, avoiding close contact with infected individuals, and regularly cleaning and disinfecting frequently touched surfaces in our environment can further reduce the risk of strep throat transmission.

Environmental Wellness:

Creating a healthy living environment plays a significant role in reducing the risk of strep throat. To prevent the spread of germs, it is important to maintain a clean and sanitized home environment. Regular cleaning of surfaces and objects, proper ventilation, and maintaining indoor air quality are essential. Avoiding exposure to environmental toxins and minimizing the use of harsh chemical cleaners can also contribute to a healthier living environment.

Social Connection and Support:

Social connection and support have a profound impact on our well-being and strep throat management. Building positive relationships and nurturing a strong support system can enhance our overall resilience and promote recovery. Reach out to loved ones, join support groups, or engage in activities that foster social connection. By cultivating social connections and building a supportive network, you can maximize your strep throat management efforts and enhance your emotional well-being during the recovery process.

Incorporating Healthy Habits Into Daily Routine:

Incorporating healthy lifestyle habits into your daily routine is crucial for effective strep throat management and long-term well-being. Consistency and sustainability are key in developing habits that will support your strep throat prevention and recovery. Start by setting realistic goals, gradually implementing healthy habits into your routine, and finding strategies to stay motivated. With time, these habits will become second nature, contributing to your overall health and reducing the risk of strep throat.

In conclusion, healthy lifestyle habits are foundational in managing and preventing strep throat. By consistently following a balanced diet, engaging in regular exercise, prioritizing adequate sleep, staying hydrated, managing stress, avoiding smoking and excessive alcohol consumption, practicing good hygiene, maintaining a healthy environment, fostering social connections, and incorporating these habits into your daily routine, you can optimize your strep throat management efforts and promote overall well-being.

Strengthening the Immune System

Strengthening the immune system is essential in managing and preventing strep throat. A robust immune system not only protects the body against infections but also promotes overall health and well-being. As a medical doctor and health and wellness coach, I emphasize the importance of a holistic approach to strengthen the immune system. Here are some key strategies to support immune health:

Proper nutrition plays a critical role in strengthening the immune system. Certain vitamins, minerals, and antioxidants are known to support immune function. Foods rich in vitamin C, such as citrus fruits and bell peppers, can enhance immune response. Zinc, found in foods like shellfish, beef, and pumpkin seeds, also supports immune health. Additionally, incorporating a variety of colorful fruits and vegetables into your diet provides a wide range of antioxidants that protect against cellular damage and promote immune system resilience.

Regular exercise is another powerful way to enhance immune system health. Physical activity increases circulation, which improves the delivery of immune cells throughout the body. It also reduces stress hormones and enhances the production of endorphins, which contribute to a stronger immune response. Aim for at least 150 minutes of moderate-intensity exercise, such as brisk walking or cycling, each week to optimize immune function.

Quality sleep is crucial for the maintenance of a strong immune system. During sleep, our bodies repair and replenish, including our immune cells. Poor sleep habits can impair immune function and increase susceptibility to infections like strep throat. Create a relaxing sleep environment, establish a regular sleep routine, and practice relaxation techniques before bed to improve sleep quality and support immune system resilience.

Chronic stress can have a detrimental effect on immune function. High levels of stress hormones can suppress the immune system, making individuals more susceptible to infections. Engaging in stress management techniques, such as deep breathing exercises, meditation, and regular physical activity, can help reduce stress levels and enhance immune system resilience. Prioritizing self-care activities, seeking support from loved ones, and practicing relaxation techniques can effectively support immune health.

In addition to lifestyle modifications, practicing good hygiene is crucial in protecting the immune system from infections. Proper handwashing techniques, covering the mouth and nose when coughing or sneezing, and regularly cleaning frequently touched surfaces can minimize the risk of strep throat transmission. Avoiding close contact with infected individuals and maintaining personal hygiene habits further contribute to immune system health.

Herbal remedies and supplements can also support immune system health. Certain herbs, such as echinacea and elderberry, have immune-boosting properties. However, it is important to consult with a healthcare professional before incorporating these remedies into your routine, as they may interact with other medications or have contraindications.

Mindfulness techniques, such as deep breathing, meditation, and yoga, promote immune system resilience by reducing stress and enhancing overall well-being. By cultivating mindfulness practices, individuals can strengthen the mind-body connection and optimize immune function.

Lifestyle modifications, such as reducing alcohol consumption, quitting smoking, and maintaining a healthy weight, are essential in supporting immune system strength. Excessive alcohol consumption and smoking can weaken the immune system, making individuals more prone to infections. Additionally, maintaining a healthy weight through regular exercise and a balanced diet can optimize immune function.

Positive relationships and social support are crucial for immune system health. Building strong interpersonal connections, fostering healthy communication, and seeking support from loved ones contribute to overall resilience and well-being. By nurturing positive relationships, individuals can enhance their immune system's ability to combat infections like strep throat.

Environmental factors also play a significant role in immune system wellness. Minimizing exposure to toxins, pollutants, and allergens can help maintain a healthy immune system. Regularly cleaning and disinfecting living spaces, maintaining proper ventilation, and minimizing the use of harsh chemical cleaners can contribute to a healthier living environment.

Taking a holistic approach to immune system strengthening is key. By addressing physical, psychological, and social aspects of well-being, individuals can promote immune system resilience and overall health. Incorporating these strategies into daily life can optimize strep throat management efforts and support long-term well-being. Remember, strengthening the immune system is a lifelong journey, and consistency is key in maintaining optimal immune health.

Chapter 7: Beyond Strep Throat: Building Resilience

Resilience in the Face of Adversity

Resilience is a concept that I hold dear to my heart, as it is an integral aspect of both physical and emotional well-being. At its core, resilience is the ability to bounce back from adversity and navigate through life's challenges with grace and strength. It is the unwavering determination to not only endure but also grow and thrive in the face of adversity. In today's world, where we are constantly bombarded with stressors and challenges, cultivating resilience has become more important than ever.

There are various factors that influence resilience, making it a dynamic and multifaceted trait. Personal attributes, such as self-confidence, optimism, and perseverance, contribute to one's resilience. Additionally, environmental factors, such as a supportive and nurturing upbringing, access to resources, and a stable social network, play a significant role in shaping our ability to cope with adversity. Moreover, the presence of a strong support system, comprising of family, friends, and professionals like myself, can provide an invaluable source of emotional support and guidance in navigating through challenging times.

A positive mindset is a powerful tool in developing resilience. The way we perceive and interpret the events in our lives has a significant impact on our emotional well-being. By consciously reframing negative thoughts and focusing on the positive aspects of a situation, we can train our minds to foster resilience. Practices like gratitude journaling, where we regularly reflect on and express gratitude for the things we have, can help shift our focus towards the positive aspects of life, even amidst adversity.

Self-compassion is another essential ingredient in building resilience. During difficult times, we often tend to be harsh and critical towards ourselves, exacerbating our emotional distress. By cultivating self-compassion, we learn to treat ourselves with kindness and understanding, providing solace when we need it the most. Engaging in self-care activities, taking time for ourselves, and practicing self-acceptance are all part of fostering self-compassion and building resilience.

Developing effective coping strategies is key to navigating through adversity. The ability to problem-solve, seek social support, and engage in self-care activities are all crucial in maintaining our emotional well-being. When faced with challenges, taking a step back, analyzing the situation, and coming up with a plan of action can provide a sense of control amidst chaos. Surrounding ourselves with a supportive network of loved ones and seeking their guidance and comfort can also be immensely helpful. Engaging in activities that bring us joy, practicing relaxation techniques, and ensuring adequate self-care can serve as healthy outlets to manage stress and build resilience.

Adaptability, the ability to embrace change, is a crucial aspect of resilience. Life is filled with uncertainties and unexpected twists, and our ability to adapt and adjust to these changes is pivotal in our ability to bounce back. Cultivating a growth mindset, which involves seeing challenges as opportunities for growth and embracing the learning process, can enable us to thrive in the face of adversity.

Building a strong support network is essential in fostering resilience. Establishing and maintaining healthy relationships can provide us with emotional support, practical assistance, and a sense of belonging. When we surround ourselves with individuals who believe in us, who uplift and encourage us, we are better equipped to face the challenges that life throws our way.

Setting realistic goals and taking consistent action towards them is another crucial aspect of resilience. By setting achievable goals and breaking them down into smaller, more manageable tasks, we enhance our sense of accomplishment and progress. Taking proactive steps towards our goals, even in the face of adversity, instills a sense of purpose and resilience.

Practicing mindfulness and stress reduction techniques are valuable tools in developing resilience. Mindfulness allows us to stay present in the moment, helping us to better navigate challenging situations without becoming overwhelmed. Techniques such as meditation, deep breathing exercises, and relaxation exercises can provide a much-needed respite in times of stress, enabling us to approach adversity with a calm and centered mind.

Adversity, although often unwelcome, can serve as a powerful catalyst for personal growth. By viewing adversity as an opportunity for development, we can transform difficult situations into moments of empowerment and self-discovery. Resilience has the potential to strengthen us and instill a profound sense of empowerment, reminding us of our own capacity to overcome adversity.

Negative thought patterns can erode our resilience and hinder our ability to bounce back from adversity. By recognizing and challenging these thought patterns, we regain control over our emotions and thoughts. Techniques such as cognitive restructuring, thought stopping, and reframing can be invaluable in changing our perspective and cultivating resilience.

Cultivating gratitude is a fundamental aspect of resilience. By practicing gratitude, we shift our focus towards the positive aspects of life, even in the face of adversity. Regularly expressing gratitude for the things we have, the people in our lives, and the lessons we have learned allows us to find solace and strength amidst challenging times.

Learning from past experiences is an important part of building resilience. Reflecting on previous challenges and identifying the strategies that have helped us bounce back can inform our actions in future adversity. By embracing the lessons learned and applying them to new situations, we enhance our resilience and ability to overcome obstacles.

Resilience is not only crucial in our personal lives but also in our relationships. The ability to adapt, communicate effectively, and resolve conflicts is vital in maintaining healthy relationships. Resilience allows us to navigate the ups and downs of relationships, fostering understanding, compassion, and mutual growth. Self-care and well-being are intrinsically linked to resilience. Prioritizing our physical, emotional, and mental well-being through activities such as exercise, healthy eating, adequate sleep, and engaging in hobbies and activities we enjoy builds the foundation for our resilience. By taking care of ourselves, we fortify our capacity to cope with challenges and adversity.

Finally, celebrating small victories and practicing self-compassion are vital components of resilience. By acknowledging our progress, no matter how small, and treating ourselves with kindness and understanding, we nurture our ability to bounce back. Self-compassion allows us to be gentle with ourselves throughout our resilience-building journey, recognizing that setbacks and struggles are part of the process.

In conclusion, resilience is a skill that can be developed and nurtured. By embracing the concept of resilience in the face of adversity, we open ourselves up to a world of possibilities. With each challenge we encounter, we have the capacity to grow stronger, more empowered, and more resilient. The path may not always be easy, but with resilience as our guiding light, we have the power to navigate through life's trials and emerge stronger on the other side.

Self-Care for Long-Term Well-being

Self-care is the cornerstone of long-term well-being. It encompasses a wide range of practices that prioritize our physical, emotional, and mental health. As a medical doctor and health and wellness coach, I have witnessed the transformative power of self-care. When we take the time to care for ourselves, we create a strong foundation for our overall well-being.

Understanding the connection between self-care and long-term well-being is crucial. Self-care practices have a profound impact on both our physical and mental health. Engaging in regular exercise, consuming a balanced diet, and getting enough rest are all fundamental aspects of physical self-care. These practices not only improve our physical health but also contribute to our mental and emotional well-being. When our bodies are nourished and energized, we are better equipped to handle the challenges and stressors of daily life.

Emotional well-being is equally important. Self-care practices such as mindfulness, journaling, and engaging in creative outlets provide us with the tools to manage our emotions and maintain a positive mindset. Taking the time to acknowledge and process our feelings allows us to develop resilience and cultivate a sense of inner peace. Self-care also involves fostering healthy relationships and seeking social support. Maintaining a strong support network helps us feel connected and supported, enhancing our emotional well-being.

Self-care is essential for maintaining a balanced and fulfilling life. By prioritizing self-care, we can ensure that all aspects of our well-being are addressed. This includes addressing our physical, emotional, social, and spiritual needs. Each of these areas is interconnected and contributes to our overall well-being. By tending to all aspects of self-care, we create a harmonious and holistic approach to our well-being.

To incorporate self-care into daily life, effective time management is crucial. Set aside dedicated time for self-care activities and prioritize them. Learn to set boundaries and say no to activities that deplete your energy. It's essential to establish a daily routine that includes self-care activities. This routine can be tailored to fit your specific needs and preferences. Even in a busy schedule, there are creative ways to practice self-care, such as taking short breaks throughout the day for deep breathing exercises or engaging in activities that bring you joy.

Creating a personalized self-care plan is vital. Assess your current self-care practices and identify areas where improvements can be made. Set realistic goals for incorporating self-care into your daily life and break them down into actionable steps. Develop a self-care plan that aligns with your individual needs and preferences. This may involve a combination of physical activities, meditation, spending time with loved ones, and engaging in hobbies that bring you joy and fulfillment.

Explore different self-care practices to find what works best for you. Physical self-care involves prioritizing exercise, nutrition, and rest. Emotional self-care includes techniques for managing stress and practicing self-compassion. Social self-care emphasizes the importance of maintaining healthy relationships and fostering connections. Spiritual self-care involves exploring practices that align with your beliefs and values.

However, some barriers may hinder self-care practices. It's important to address guilt or feelings of selfishness related to prioritizing self-care. Understand that taking care of yourself is essential for your well-being and enables you to better support those around you. Seek support from others in your self-care journey. Surround yourself with people who uplift and encourage you, and share your self-care goals and challenges with them.

Regularly evaluate and adapt your self-care plan. Monitor your progress and identify areas that may need more attention. Celebrate your successes and learn from any setbacks. Self-care is not a one-size-fits-all approach and may need to be adjusted based on various life stages and circumstances. Adapt your self-care practices to fit your changing needs or health conditions. During challenging times and transitions, self-care becomes even more critical.

Consistency is key in maintaining self-care for long-term well-being. Make self-care a lifelong practice and integrate it into your daily life. Create a support network that can help you stay accountable and motivated. Embrace self-care as the foundation of a balanced and fulfilling life, knowing that by caring for yourself, you are cultivating resilience and well-being. In the journey of life, self-care is the compass that guides us to a state of holistic health and long-lasting well-being.

Mindfulness and Gratitude

In this chapter, let's explore the powerful combination of mindfulness and gratitude, and how they can contribute to your overall well-being, particularly in the context of managing strep throat.

Mindfulness, the practice of bringing one's attention to the present moment without judgment, can have profound effects on reducing stress and improving mental clarity. By cultivating a state of mindfulness, you can become more attuned to the sensations and experiences in your body, ultimately enhancing your emotional well-being. In the midst of dealing with strep throat, practicing mindfulness can be especially beneficial as it helps you focus on the present moment, rather than dwelling on the discomfort or worrying about the future.

Integrating gratitude into your daily life can also play a significant role in promoting well-being. Gratitude involves recognizing and appreciating the positive aspects of one's life, no matter how small. By consciously cultivating a grateful mindset, you can increase feelings of happiness, satisfaction, and contentment. When facing the challenges of strep throat, gratitude can offer a respite from the physical discomfort and emotional strain, reminding you of the positive aspects of your life and promoting a more positive mindset.

So, how can you incorporate mindfulness and gratitude into your daily life? Here are a few practical strategies:

1. Start with mindfulness exercises: Begin your day with a simple mindfulness practice, such as deep breathing or a body scan. Take a few moments to connect with your breath and bring your attention to the sensations in your body. Throughout the day, pause and check in with yourself, noticing any thoughts or emotions without judgment.

2. Keep a gratitude journal: Set aside a few minutes each day to write down three things you are grateful for. They could be small moments, acts of kindness, or things that bring you joy. Reflecting

on these moments of gratitude can help shift your focus towards the positive aspects of your life and promote a sense of well-being, even in the face of strep throat.

3. Practice gratitude meditation: Dedicate a few minutes each day to a gratitude meditation. Find a quiet space, close your eyes, and bring your attention to the things you are grateful for. Let feelings of gratitude fill your heart and mind, directing your attention to the positive aspects of your life. This practice can be particularly helpful in fostering a sense of calm and peace, even amidst the discomfort of strep throat.

Now, you might be wondering, what does science say about mindfulness and gratitude? Research has shown that both practices have positive effects on physical health, immune function, and psychological well-being. When it comes to strep throat, incorporating mindfulness and gratitude into your treatment regimen can complement medical interventions and support your overall well-being.

For further guidance and support on your mindfulness and gratitude journey, there are numerous resources available. Books, apps, and online courses can provide you with the tools and techniques to deepen your practice and integrate mindfulness and gratitude into your daily life.

Remember, consistency and patience are key when practicing mindfulness and gratitude. Treat them as lifelong practices and integrate them into your daily routine. By embracing mindfulness and gratitude, you can cultivate resilience, promote healing, and experience profound positive changes in your life, even in the midst of managing strep throat.

Thriving Beyond Strep Throat

Introduction to Thriving Beyond Strep Throat

As a healthcare professional who believes in the power of holistic healing, I am here to guide you on your journey to thriving beyond strep throat. This segment will delve into the concept of embracing a holistic approach to your health and well-being, empowering you to take an active role in your recovery journey. By embracing holistic healthcare practices, lifestyle modifications, and self-care techniques, you will not only overcome the challenges of strep throat, but also find newfound strength and resilience within yourself.

Overcoming the Challenges of Strep Throat

Living with strep throat can be physically and emotionally challenging. The painful sore throat, difficulty swallowing, and fatigue can make even the simplest tasks feel overwhelming. However, I am here to assure you that you have the power to rise above these challenges and emerge stronger than ever. By viewing this condition as an opportunity for personal growth and transformation, you can overcome the physical and emotional difficulties associated with strep throat. Remember, you are not defined by your illness, but rather by your ability to overcome it.

Embracing Holistic Healing

Holistic healing is a practice that focuses on addressing not only the physical symptoms of an illness but also the psychological and social aspects of your well-being. When it comes to strep throat, it is crucial to seek out healthcare providers who understand the importance of a holistic approach. By addressing all aspects of your health, including lifestyle modifications, nutrition, stress management, and psychological well-being, you will be on the path to recovery and thriving beyond strep throat. Remember, your journey to wellness encompasses more than just the eradication of the bacteria; it involves taking care of your whole self.

Finding Meaning in the Healing Journey

Every experience, including strep throat, has the potential to teach us valuable lessons and offer growth opportunities. By reflecting on your experiences and finding meaning in your healing journey, you can discover a newfound sense of purpose and fulfillment. Take the time to evaluate your priorities, reexamine your relationships, and embrace a more fulfilling and purposeful life. Strep throat may have brought you to your knees, but it is up to you to rise above it and embrace the lessons it has to offer.

Nurturing Physical and Emotional Well-being

During your recovery process from strep throat, it is essential to prioritize both your physical and emotional well-being. Take care of your body by nourishing it with healthy, nutrient-rich foods, getting adequate rest, and engaging in gentle exercise. Additionally, seek out emotional support through therapy, support groups, or connections with loved ones. Remember, you are not alone in this journey, and by nurturing both your physical and emotional well-being, you will flourish beyond strep throat.

Cultivating Resilience and Adaptability

Strep throat may have disrupted your life, but it is an opportunity to cultivate resilience and adaptability. Embrace challenges as opportunities for growth, and approach your recovery with a mindset of resilience. Be open to adapting to your changing circumstances and find new ways to thrive beyond strep throat. By developing these qualities, you will not only conquer strep throat but also be better prepared to face any future obstacles with confidence and grace.

Building a Supportive Network

Surrounding yourself with a supportive network is vital to your recovery and thriving beyond strep throat. Seek out healthcare providers who offer a holistic approach and can guide you on your healing journey. Additionally, connect with friends, family, or support groups who understand and empathize with your experience. Building a network of positive, understanding individuals will provide the emotional support necessary to navigate the ups and downs of your recovery journey.

Celebrating Successes and Milestones

Don't forget to celebrate your progress along the way. No matter how small, each step towards full recovery is an achievement worth acknowledging. Set achievable goals and celebrate when you reach them. By recognizing and appreciating your successes and milestones, you will foster a sense of confidence and motivation to continue thriving beyond strep throat.

Embracing Mind-Body Connection

The mind-body connection plays a vital role in thriving beyond strep throat. Practices such as meditation, mindfulness, and visualization can help you harness the power of your thoughts and emotions for healing. Consider integrating practices like yoga, tai chi, and breathwork into your routine to promote overall well-being. These practices will not only support your physical healing but also foster emotional resilience, helping you thrive in the face of strep throat.

Inspiring Others Through Your Personal Journey

Finally, use your personal journey of thriving beyond strep throat to inspire and support others facing similar challenges. Share your experiences and become an advocate for holistic healthcare. By sharing your story, you have the power to create a ripple effect of hope and empowerment within your community. Remember, your journey is not just about your own healing; it is about supporting and uplifting others on their paths to recovery.

In conclusion, thriving beyond strep throat is not just about eradicating the bacteria from your body. It is about embracing a holistic approach to your health and well-being, nurturing your physical and emotional self, and finding meaning in the healing journey. By cultivating resilience, adapting to challenges, building a supportive network, celebrating successes, embracing the mind-body connection, and inspiring others, you will not only overcome strep throat but also emerge as a stronger, healthier, and more fulfilled individual. Together, let's thrive beyond strep throat and lead lives filled with wellness, purpose, and joy.

Milton Keynes UK
Ingram Content Group UK Ltd.
UKHW020652200923
429044UK00014B/358